EDUCATING COMPETENT AND HUMANE PHYSICIANS

Educating Competent and Humane Physicians

HUGH C. HENDRIE AND
CAMILLE LLOYD

EDITORS

INDIANA UNIVERSITY PRESS
Bloomington and Indianapolis

The figure in chapter 3 is reprinted by permission of the publisher from
"The Timing of Psychiatric Consultation
in the General Hospital and Length of Hospital Stay,"
by John Lyons, Jeffrey Hammer, James Strain, and George Fulop,
General Hospital Psychiatry, vol. 8, p. 160.
Copyright 1986 by Elsevier Science Publishing Co., Inc.

The paper used in this publication meets the minimum requirements of American
National Standard for Information Sciences—Permanence of Paper for Printed
Library Materials, ANSI Z39.48-1984.

Manufactured in the United States of America

Library of Congress Cataloging-in-Publication Data

Educating competent and humane physicians / Hugh C. Hendrie, Camille
    Lloyd, editors.
        p.   cm.
    Dedicated to the memory of Nancy Roeske.
    ISBN 0-253-32725-3 (alk paper)
    1. Medical education—Psychological aspects.   2. Medical
education—Philosophy.   3. Physician and patient.   4. Roeske, Nancy A., 1928–
1986.   I. Hendrie, Hugh C.   II. Lloyd, Camille   III. Roeske, Nancy A., 1928–
1986.
    [DNLM: 1. Clinical Competence.   2. Education, Medical.
3. Humanism.   W 18 E2364]
    R737.E28   1990
    610'.71'1—dc20
    DNLM/DLC
    for Library of Congress   89-45473
                                                                CIP

1 2 3 4 5   94 93 92 91 90

CONTENTS

PREFACE
> *Hugh C. Hendrie and Camille Lloyd* / vii

TRIBUTES TO NANCY C. A. ROESKE
> *Martha Kirkpatrick, Howard P. Rome* / x

CONTRIBUTORS / xiii

Part One Biotechnical Competence Is Not Enough: The Need for Humane and Psychosocially Sophisticated Physicians / 1

1 Facts and Values in Medical Education
The Role of Human Relationships in Health, Illness, and Disease
> *Herbert Weiner* / 3

2 Symptoms without Signs
Somatic Presentation of Psychiatric Illness
> *Geoffrey G. Lloyd* / 24

3 Psychiatry in Medicine
Cost-Effectiveness Studies
> *James J. Strain, George Fulop, Jeffrey S. Hammer, and John S. Lyons* / 35

4 Communication
The Key to Becoming Competent and Humane Physicians
> *Leah J. Dickstein* / 54

5 The Ideal Physician
Requisite Attitudes, Knowledge, and Skills
> *Hugh C. Hendrie* / 72

Part Two Current Medical Education and the Development of Humaneness / 81

6 The Impact of the Educational System on the Development of the Modern Hippocrates
> *Roger J. Bulger* / 83

7 Facilitating Humaneness in Medical Students and Residents
> *Camille Lloyd and Ann Gateley* / 94

**Part Three   Toward a More Humane Medicine: Lessons from the
Past and Recent Innovations in Medical Education**
/ 115

8   Women's Contribution to Medical Education
A Nineteenth-Century Case Study
Regina Morantz-Sanchez / 117

9   Innovations in Medical Education
Enhancing Humanism through the Educational Process
*Maggie Moore-West, Martha Regan-Smith, Allen Dietrich, and
Donald O. Kollisch* / 128

10   Promoting the Adaptation and Coping of Pediatric Residents
Morris Green / 175

11   Reducing Stress in Medical Oncology House Officers
A Preliminary Report of a Prospective Intervention Study
Kathryn M. Kash and Jimmie C. Holland / 183

Part Four   Physician Training: A Sociocultural Perspective
/ 197

12   Training in Caring Competence
The Perennial Problem in North American Medical Education
Renée C. Fox / 199

INDEX / 217

Preface

HUGH C. HENDRIE AND CAMILLE LLOYD

This volume intends to address issues of medical education, particularly the necessity for and the current efforts in training physicians who have the professional competence and personal qualities required to practice comprehensive and humane health care and the barriers that exist within the medical school structure to the attainment of this goal.

While many of these issues have been discussed previously both in the professional and lay press, it is the editors' belief that the present volume offers several advantages. It documents advances in both the psychosocial and neurobiological sciences that explain why familiarity with the basic biological sciences as currently taught is not sufficient by itself for the practice of medicine. Rather than call attention to the current general discontent with medical education's failure to develop the most humane practitioner, the book identifies specific aspects of the educational process that adversely impact or impede the desired compassion and psychosocial sophistication needed in medical practitioners. It also provides a comprehensive review of the empirical literature suggesting that the current medical education process can be detrimental to both the humanity of medical trainees and their sense of well-being. Finally, it brings together valuable information about innovative approaches to medical education that attempt to address these deficiencies. Much of the information about such innovative efforts has been previously available only anecdotally or informally in meetings of medical educators. The collection of such material into one volume will facilitate a thorough discussion of the issues involved and will hopefully advance efforts to educate truly humane physicians.

The first of the book's four parts is devoted to presentations in five chapters of the evidence that awareness of psychosocial factors is crucial in understanding the pathogenesis of disease and illness behavior and that interpersonal and communication skills are vital requirements to practice medicine and can affect illness outcomes. A review of the attitudes, knowledge, and skills that should be acquired by physicians in addition to those already acquired in biomedical training in order to provide competent and humane clinical care is also presented.

In part two, the structure and functioning of the medical school setting is analyzed with respect to its impact on the development of humanistic qualities in medical trainees and its effect on the well-being of medical students and residents. In the chapters in this section it is noted that there is an analogy between the faculty-student relationship and the doctor-patient relationship: a caring relationship in the former presages compassion in the latter.

Part three details selected efforts to sensitize physicians-in-training to the human aspects of medical practice. The first chapter of this part places current efforts in this regard in historical context by returning to the nineteenth century to describe how women's medical colleges and early prominent women physicians addressed these concerns. The second chapter of part three provides a valuable summary of recent innovations in medical education which, among other aims, have attempted to humanize medical practice. The chapter also provides preliminary assessments of the efficacy of such innovations. The two other chapters of this part describe programmatic efforts aimed at reducing stress among house staff and providing them with a more humane setting in which to work.

In the final part, Renée Fox provides a fitting summation of the themes raised previously in the book as she places in a psychosocial context the perennial problem of providing training in caring competence for physicians and discusses some solutions.

This volume is dedicated to the memory of Nancy Roeske, Professor of Psychiatry at Indiana University School of Medicine, who died in April 1986. She was concerned throughout her distinguished professional career about the socialization process of the health professional and the appropriate environment for medical education. Tributes from two of her colleagues are included.

The book is addressed primarily to those involved in the education of physicians. The editors anticipate, however, that because of the breadth of the topics and the general concern about health-related matters, it will also appeal to medical students, students of the health-related disciplines, and the interested lay public.

ACKNOWLEDGMENT

The editors gratefully acknowledge the tireless secretarial and organizational help provided by Mrs. Francine Bray in preparing this volume.

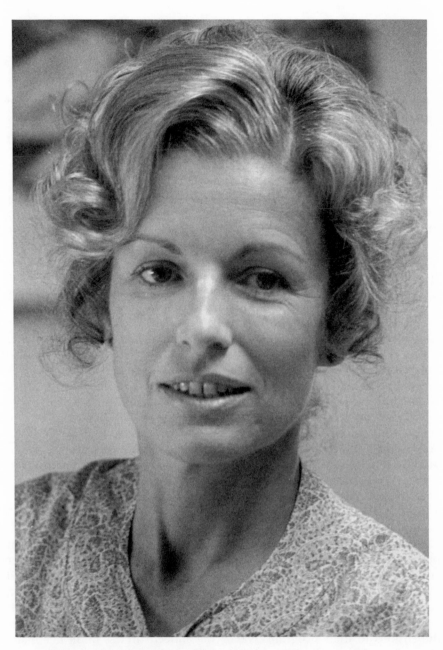

NANCY C. A. ROESKE, M.D.
APRIL 17, 1928–APRIL 21, 1986

Tributes to Nancy C. A. Roeske

I am writing this brief tribute to Nancy Roeske on my way home from my second American Psychiatric Association Annual Meeting without Nancy. Last year, 1986, Nancy and I talked on the phone to plan our rooming together at the upcoming Annual Meeting. That was just days before her sudden death. I knew, of course, that she had been ill. I knew she was continuing to work in her thorough, determined, and consistent way, writing reports two days after surgery, working at her office or at home despite the enervating and demoralizing effects of chemotherapy. And I knew this might be the last time we would share midnight thoughts about strategies to increase the involvement of women psychiatrists at the policy-making level of the APA, or about her passionate involvement with the Indiana School for the Blind, or about our families, our own ambitions and hopes and disappointments. Nancy was a very ambitious person, and she was ambitious for all of us who came under her sway.

I met Nancy when I was a member of the APA Task Force on Women. Nancy was the chairperson. I had served on many committees, as member and as chairperson, but watching Nancy I realized I had never understood the role of the chair in setting an achievable agenda, defining a work product, and facilitating (not dictating) the means to effect that product. Nancy was a masterly mistress of our proceedings. The Task Force produced documents on supervision and teaching (or the lack of it) by and about women in psychiatric residencies, on psychiatric journals' policies, and on the composition of editorial boards and review boards. We found out how much longer it took women to climb the academic ladder, how few women researchers received grants, and why. We learned that this changed dramatically when women were added to the review boards of granting agencies. Due to the success of the Task Force it became a standing APA Committee. Nancy continued to promote the cause of women in the APA. She believed that both the future of women psychiatrists and the future of humanistic trends in psychiatry depended on attention to the broader education and socialization of residents. Toward this end she worked tirelessly (and against a variety of obstacles) to develop and publish a curriculum on male and female development that could act as an impetus and model for faculty or residents hoping to add a course in gender dimensions to their program. Nancy was indeed tireless in all her many efforts, sometimes unreasonably so, as when she delayed a hysterectomy that was clearly necessary until it was forced on her as a life-saving emergency. She then made use of the experience to investigate and write about women's reactions to hysterectomy.

Nancy was dedicated to the medical identity of psychiatry. She worked vigorously in the AMA as well as the APA. Her loyalty to medicine as the noblest profession was deeply embedded in her pride and devotion to her mother, an obstetrician/gynecologist. Thus, for her, medical tradition had always had a maternal core and blended suitably into her feminine identity. She was unburdened by the conflicts surrounding the choice of medicine as a career, the fear of losing one's "femininity" by joining a "male" profession, or the fear that a medical career and a family life were mutually exclusive. She hoped to encourage women to seek medicine as a most legitimate career for the use of their feminine interests, the caring and nurturing of those in need, the interest in and respect for individual development and individual suffering, the priority of personal pain over abstract principles. Nancy knew that the scientific ideal of medicine, however necessary and creative, must be balanced by such humanistic ideals. I deeply valued her as a model of the best of both these traditions and of the tradition of friendship that endures over time and distance.

—*Martha Kirkpatrick*

As I think about Nancy Roeske, my thoughts consist of a patterned mosaic. Each of the tessera, while different, is wonderfully blended with all others to produce a luminous composition. Death confers a unique perspective. It allows one to see with biographical insight. In this way, one is able to view the many works of a life as reflecting an underlying theme of compassionate caring.

Nancy's illustrious career seen in this light is another reflection of her entire life. Her intensity was born of a life lived to the full with a larger than usual share of poignant stressful experiences. Typically, she used these in a way that converted their misfortunes to riches. The result was an annealing process, for the pain of their stress was distilled and thereby converted into what can only be called compassionate empathy. She was zealous in her devotion. This spirit is the nectar of humanism.

Most persons knew of her ardent feminism. Indeed, she was unceasing in her struggles for women's rights. But this was just another facet of her humanism that demanded equal rights for all according to their capacities. She saw discrimination as anathema. Also, she was realistic. Therefore, people as a whole were judged and rewarded on the basis of their needs as persons deserving of succor, guidance, and opportunities to fulfill to the utmost their capacities. It is this, above all else, that ennobles her life work; thereby the needy mentally ill, as well as the lame, the halt and the blind, were by their disablements entitled to the best that medicine had to offer in concert with the lay community, whose largesse far extended beyond financial support. She saw this as the essence of unstinted charity—much more than mere giving.

Because she was a recipient of a rare form of education that coupled caring with instruction, her life to the end replicated the ways she had learned to teach. Of course, this endeared her to her pupils, who became her friends, and also brought her admiration from her colleagues. It must be said that there were those who resented her forceful presentations. It is forever thus in human affairs. In our talks, Nancy knew that her zealous endeavor created obstacles that she saw as resistance, being the perceptive psychiatrist she was. One must deal with this kind of oppositional behavior as if it were akin to resistance in a psychotherapeutic encounter. Sooner or later it would be transformed by educational insights into a better understanding of the personal derivatives of repressed antecedent problems. Nancy handled these situations with her customary aplomb.

Gallantry—that rare aspect of sublimation—is ultimately recognized as a consequence of a rich life fully lived and examined. As the wise Socrates held long ago, an examined life does not end with a period but with an . . .

Nancy Arnold Roeske, M.D.
RIP

—Howard P. Rome

Contributors

ROGER J. BULGER, M.D.
President, Association of Academic
  Health Centers and Clinical
  Professor of Medicine
11 DuPont Circle N.W.
Washington, D.C.

LEAH J. DICKSTEIN, M.D.
Professor, Department of Psychiatry
Associate Dean for Student Affairs
University of Louisville School of
  Medicine
Louisville, Kentucky

ALLEN DIETRICH, M.D.
Clinical Associate Professor
Department of Community and Family
  Medicine & Director of
  Undergraduate Family Medical
  Education
Dartmouth Medical School
Hanover, New Hampshire

RENÉE C. FOX, PH.D.
Annenberg Professor of the Social
  Sciences
Department of Sociology
University of Pennsylvania
Philadelphia, Pennsylvania

GEORGE FULOP, M.D.
Clinical Assistant Professor
Department of Psychiatry
Mount Sinai School of Medicine
New York, New York

ANN GÀTELEY, M.D.
Associate Director of House Staff &
  Assistant Professor, Department of
  Internal Medicine
The University of Texas Health Science
  Center
Houston, Texas

MORRIS GREEN, M.D.
Perry W. Lesh Professor of Pediatrics
Department of Pediatrics
Indiana University School of Medicine
Indianapolis, Indiana

JEFFREY S. HAMMER, M.D.
Director, Quality Assurance
Veterans Administration Medical
  Center
Los Angeles, California

HUGH C. HENDRIE, M.B., CH.B.
Chairman & Albert E. Sterne Professor
Department of Psychiatry
Indiana University School of Medicine
Indianapolis, Indiana

JIMMIE C. HOLLAND, M.D.
Chief, Psychiatry Service
Memorial Sloan-Kettering Cancer
  Center
Professor, Department of Psychiatry
Cornell University Medical College
New York, New York

KATHRYN M. KASH, PH.D.
Clinical Assistant Attending
  Psychologist
Psychiatry Service
Memorial Sloan-Kettering Cancer
  Center
New York, New York

MARTHA KIRKPATRICK, M.D.
A Medical Corporation
988 Bluegrass Lane
Los Angeles, California

DONALD O. KOLLISCH, M.D.
Assistant Professor
Department of Community and Family
  Medicine
Dartmouth Medical School
Hanover, New Hampshire

GEOFFREY G. LLOYD, M.D., F.R.C.P.,
  F.R.C.PSYCH.
Consultant Psychiatrist
Royal Free Hospital
London, England

CAMILLE LLOYD, PH.D.
Director, Student Counseling Service
Associate Professor of Psychiatry

xiii

The University of Texas Health Science
  Center
Houston, Texas

JOHN S. LYONS, M.D.
Associate Professor
Department of Psychiatry
Northwestern Memorial Hospital
Chicago, Illinois

MAGGIE MOORE-WEST, PH.D.
Research Associate Professor
Department of Community & Family
  Medicine & Director of Educational
  Research and Educational Evaluation
Office of Academic and Student Affairs
Dartmouth Medical School
Hanover, New Hampshire

REGINA MORANTZ-SANCHEZ, PH.D.
Professor
Department of History
University of California
Los Angeles, California

MARTHA REGAN-SMITH, M.D.
Associate Professor of Medicine and
  Assistant Dean for Clinical Education
Dartmouth Medical School
Hanover, New Hampshire

HOWARD P. ROME, M.D.
Emeritus Professor of Psychiatry
Mayo Graduate School of Medicine
Rochester, Minnesota

JAMES J. STRAIN, M.D.
Professor of Clinical Psychiatry
The Mount Sinai Medical Center
New York, New York

HERBERT WEINER, M.D., DR. MED.
  (HON.)
Professor of Psychiatry & Biobehavioral
  Sciences
School of Medicine
University of California
Los Angeles, California

EDUCATING COMPETENT AND HUMANE PHYSICIANS

Part One

Biotechnical Competence Is Not Enough

THE NEED FOR HUMANE AND PSYCHOSOCIALLY SOPHISTICATED PHYSICIANS

Part one is devoted to presentations of the evidence that awareness of psychosocial factors is crucial in understanding the pathogenesis of disease and illness behavior and that interpersonal and communication skills are vital requirements to practice medicine and can effect illness outcome.

Herbert Weiner reminds us that ill health and disease are not necessarily synonymous and from this discussion emphasizes that the appropriate concern for physicians should be patients, not disease. He reviews the now extensive literature that implicates psychosocial factors in disease pathogenesis and outcome and discusses some possible explanatory mechanisms. In view of this evidence, he argues that the role human relationships play in health and disease can be presented in as factual a manner as the data from any other discipline and that its study is crucial to the education of physicians.

Geoffrey Lloyd reviews the studies demonstrating that about 30 percent of patients who attend primary care clinics present with somatic symptoms for which there is no organic pathology. He describes the presenting symptoms of the so-called somaticizers and differentiates organically based from psychically based symptoms. He reviews the underlying psychiatric syndromes that may exist in these patients, presents some explanatory hypotheses, and discusses possible management techniques.

James Strain and colleagues review the relatively new but burgeoning evidence that psychosocial intervention can influence illness outcome and be cost-effective. He emphasizes the necessity, however, of more carefully controlled studies to elucidate the putative mechanisms underlying the therapeutic effectiveness of these interventions.

Leah Dickstein emphasizes the necessity for the development of good communication skills for physicians. Yet there is considerable evidence that these skills are not always present in physicians and, worse still, are not at present well taught in medical schools. She discusses factors in the medical school educational system that may vitiate the development of good communication skills and reviews some innovative approaches to the teaching of essential interpersonal skills.

In the last chapter of this part an overview is presented of the attitudes, knowledge, and skills that should be acquired by physicians in addition to those already assessed in biomedical training in order to provide competent and humane clinical care. These include the qualities of compassion, integrity, and respect; the knowledge derived from the behavioral and population-based sciences; and the skills necessary to develop good communication with patients and to continue to acquire and access knowledge in this age of information explosion.

ONE

Facts and Values in Medical Education

The Role of Human Relationships in Health, Illness, and Disease

HERBERT WEINER

Nancy Roeske devoted her professional life to what she most valued: the education of humane medical students and physicians, so as to make them the agents of improved patient care and especially of the care of the most disadvantaged patients. In this task, she was aided by her personal attributes, moral seriousness and dedication: she personified the humane and caring physician for all but the most obtuse students to see and to model themselves after. The importance of learning by role modeling has recently been lost sight of in medical education, buried under the mass of facts students are expected to learn.

Facts and Values

Medical educators treat facts and values as if they lay at opposite poles. After all, facts are absolute, objective, verifiable, impersonal, and material. Facts do not lie. They count. They are there for anyone to see. They are teachable. Disagreement about the truth of a fact can be resolved in a determinate way. Whether a bacterium is Gram positive or negative is a question of fact; whatever the answer may be, it is clear and unambiguous.

Values are relative, subjective, unprovable, spiritual, pluralistic, and personal. They do not seem to count. Values may distort. It is hard to refute them and to teach them. Evaluative disagreement may be unresolvable: whether Mozart's Requiem is more beautiful than Verdi's is a matter of opinion and taste to which anyone in a democracy is entitled.

If the polarity of fact and value exists as a stereotype in medicine, why

3

do we value facts so, and why are we taught to evaluate them? Facts and values are not poles apart but are closely intertwined. The demarcation of facts rests squarely on considerations of values (e.g., whether they are correct, or relevant to the practice of medicine or not). Conversely, evaluations (should one terminate the life of a desperately ill patient or not?) are riddled with considerations of fact.

The highest praise accorded to an experiment is that it is elegant. How can facts be aesthetic, if beauty is in the eye of the beholder? Yet theoretical physicists unblushingly test theories by their simplicity and beauty. But in contrast to the tenets of biomedical scientists, physicists believe in the beauty of a theory. They can define beauty: beauty is symmetry, mathematically related to the concept of invariance. Einstein (Hoffman 1972) stated that the ultimate test of a physical theory was not only its correctness but also its simple beauty.

Therefore, facts are neither independent from, nor indifferent to, human concerns and judgments. We impose the criteria and enforce the standards for what counts as a fact. We stipulate: "whatever is, is physical," or "no mind without brain." In effect we decree that whatever fails to satisfy our standards does not have what it takes to be a fact. At the same time we arrange our standards to be met. If we state that "whatever is, is physical" in medicine, then all the symptoms of illness and disease—its main subject matter—must have a material (physical) explanation. And indeed, that is the tradition begun by Morgagni and carried through by Bichat and Virchow. If we maintain that the "heart is a pump" and "the brain is a computer" then the parts of the body, or the body itself, is a machine (albeit, according to Claude Bernard, a living one). These are the stated facts of medicine—they are material and mechanical.

Of course, we grudgingly accord some room in medicine for "compassion" and being humane (Mellinkoff 1984). The irony and inconsistency of this position is never stated: why should a physician be compassionate or humane to a machine? Yet we are told that compassion or humaneness cannot be defined, therefore it cannot be taught systematically, any more than one can systematically teach honesty to politicians. In fact, facts about human beings are soft—not hard, measurable, objective. To be a compassionate or humane physician is self-understood, but one cannot prove that such a physician makes much difference to treatment. So, certain values in medicine are axiomatic, but they are not objective or measurable. Like mathematical axioms they are not provable. The principle value-laden axiom in medicine is that human life is sacrosanct. No hard facts can be summoned up to support it. The only evidence for it is of a negative kind: physicians who do not hold to the axiom have contributed to some of the darkest chapters in history.

Given that only a certain class of facts are taught in medical schools, I shall hold that the very material that is usually classified as value-laden and soft—the central role of relationships—can be taught factually.

Teaching about the Importance of Human Relationships

Value judgments about the nature of facts continue to lead medical educators astray. Such pronouncements reveal prejudice and ignorance about a body of factual information central to the theory and practice of medicine: educators contend that these facts are anecdotal—a pejorative term for an observation. Facts, they contend, must be quantitative, or we must know the mechanism by which bereavement alters the level of a hormone or of an immunological parameter: the correlation does not count as a fact, only the mechanism does! But as the ensuing review will show, such facts about the relevance for medicine of knowledge about the central role played by human relationships in health, illness, and disease exist. Our past ignorance about mechanism stems from our still rudimentary understanding of the function of the brain in mediating the recorded effects.

In the past thirty years, a substantial and verified clinical and research literature has grown up to support the belief that human relationships are crucial to the maintenance of health. A corollary of that statement is that disruptions of relationships are conducive to changes in mood, behavior, the onset of illness and disease, and even death, but not in all persons; increases in mortality following bereavement occur only at certain ages and in men but not in women.

The observation that good relationships play a role in the maintenance or restoration of health should not be surprising: in every culture sick persons turn to others for help, support, advice, and cure. If it were not so the roles of physician and nurse would not have survived.

In the recent past, analytic animal studies have observed the role of mothers as important regulators of the behavior and bodily functions of their young. These studies have also thrown light on the nature of the mother-infant bond, which has a number of components, each of which acts through a different input channel of the young animal to regulate separate bodily functions and behavior. The long-term effects of disrupting the bond are to predispose the young animal to disease processes, especially when it is later challenged.

It is not surprising that clinical observers, as well as more formal retrospective, prospective, and cross-sectional studies, have indicated that bereavement by death or other partings plays a crucial role in the onset of illness and disease.

THE EFFECTS OF SEPARATION AND LOSS

Separation or bereavement may be especially poignant for adults if they recapitulate a loss in chidhood. The usual or the aberrant responses to loss may also occur when prized attributes (beauty, dignity, youth, strength, income, wealth, intelligence, skills, memory, ideals, occupations, body functions or parts, health and the sense of well-being) are lost. Loss may be anticipated and mourning may be over by the time the actual loss occurs.

Physicians are confronted daily with dying patients, their bereaved relatives, or patients who have lost some critical mental or bodily function or body part. Right now, physicians are faced with the unprecedented disaster of acquired immune deficiency syndrome (AIDS). Once the syndrome is acquired its mortality is 100 percent. The HIV virus and its consequences have struck terror into the heart of health professionals and generated prejudice in their minds. A sense of helplessness and even reluctance about caring for the victims of AIDS pervades health professionals. For its (often young) victims the disease is a tragic, poignant, and deeply sad experience. The physician preparing to care for these and other dying patients had better be thoroughly acquainted with the experience of grief, the mourning process, and its expression and observations.

Grief and the mourning process have been thoroughly described (Lindemann 1944; Bowlby 1963; Parkes 1970, 1971; Raphael 1975, 1977; Paulley 1982; Brown and Stoudemire 1983). The process normally goes through three well-characterized phases: shock and protest; despair, realization, and grief; and resolution.

The phase of resolution may never occur. More seriously, the normal mourning process may be replaced by pathological grief reactions, which may begin in the immediate aftermath of the loss or may be delayed in onset. This aberrant form of mourning consists of a complex mixture of love, longing, and need for the lost person mixed with hatred, anger, and bitterness. Feelings of vengefulness produce a cascade of anguish, guilt, and fears of retribution and the need to make amends, or pleas for forgiveness. Pathological mourning can be anticipatory: it may also occur in childhood, and is often again induced in adulthood by seemingly trivial losses (Bowlby 1963; Paulley 1982) or in persons incapable of expressing feelings (Lindemann 1944). Pathological mourning occurs when certain kinds of people—those who rely on others and are not capable of mature relationships—are bereft of the other person by unexpected or unusual circumstances such as murder, suicide, or disappearance (Parkes 1971; Raphael 1977). The survivor's guilt stems from the belief that he or she wittingly or unwittingly drove the partner away (or to suicide).

Pathological mourning is a major risk factor for depression and/or suicide, for the acquisition of the departed's symptoms and behaviors, and for a life of bitterness, social isolation, and suffering. The mourner may distract himself or herself with restless overactivity in order to remain oblivious to the profound sense of loss and the cascade of painful feelings it has engendered.

Grief and pathological mourning need not be expressed at all following a loss. The onset may be delayed; symptoms may occur only on key anniversaries or, as noted, after seemingly trivial losses, and be associated with the onset of disease. Survivors may deny the death of a relative and live in a make-believe world. Some people disguise their grief in chronic anger or become touchy or impassive. They may be incapable of experiencing or expressing feelings.

Major depressive symptoms may have their onset with a latent period of weeks or months after a loss or bereavement. In such patients, causal connections between the event and the illness cannot be made, and they deny that they feel sad. Or delayed grief reactions may be transmuted into pain and hyperventilation syndromes of a variety of kinds.

Following the death of a relative, some survivors, rather than feeling grief, remarry quickly (after a spouse has died) or try to replace a dead child by becoming pregnant or by adopting one. Sooner or later they become symptomatic if they have never grieved their immediate bereavement.

Because of their age-inappropriate psychological makeup, those who mourn pathologically are particularly in need of encouragement, ventilation of their complex feelings, and advice (Raphael 1975).

EXPERIMENTAL STUDIES ON SEPARATION

Observations on grief and the mourning process have been made and confirmed by many clinicians in the twentieth century. They were given their initial impetus by Sigmund Freud.

In the past thirty-five years the behavioral observations made on humans have been complemented and supplemented by experimental work on other mammals. The phases of grief outlined above can be observed in the behavior of separated rats, dogs, and monkeys. But it remained for Hofer (1981) and his co-workers to combine behavioral and physiological observations in experiments on rats.

Hofer (1981, 1982) and Weiner (1982) have pointed out that both in animals and man, separation can be divided into two phases. The acute protest phase is seen both in human infants and adults. Out of this phase a chronic background of disturbance develops. In the adult, the protest phase seen in the infant corresponds in time and quality to the phase of shock, despair, and realization.

We know a great deal more about the physiological changes in young animals following separation than about those occurring in adults. Young animals show a variety of psychobiological responses to being prematurely separated from their mothers. A careful analysis of the effects of separation indicates that it is not a global experience. In fact, the experience of separation is highly discriminated because each behavioral or physiological system of the infant normally responds to a separate input from the mother and her infant; separation terminates them. Rats separated at fifteen days of age, show increased motor activity in the form of self-grooming, rearing up, moving about, and squealing. These behaviors are suppressed by the physical presence of the mother, who provides warmth and tactile stimulation. These young animals are unable to regulate their body temperatures;

when it falls their activity declines. In separated rats with low body temperature the levels of catecholamines, protein, and nucleoprotein in their brains fall (Hofer 1981).

Specific areas of the infant rats' bodies are stimulated by the mother. She licks the back of the infants' neck. She picks them up by the scruff of the neck. When the infants are not stimulated at this site, levels of growth hormone and ornithine decarboxylase in the heart and brain rapidly decline (Butler et al. 1978; Kuhn et al. 1978; Evoniuk et al. 1979).

The touch of the nipple on the infant's lips increases nonnutritive sucking, which is diminished in the mother's absence. The sense of smell is critical to the attachment of the infant to the nipple because the areolar glands appear to produce a chemically unidentified pheromone that attracts the infant. This substance is under the control of oxytocin, which in turn is released in the mother rat by suckling. When this pheromone is washed off or the olfactory epithelium of the infant is destroyed, the infant does not attach itself to the nipple and begins to demonstrate the motor behaviors seen in separated rats.

Nutritive suckling in infants declines in separated rats and is restored when milk distends the stomach. The heart and respiratory rate of baby rats falls 30 percent within two to four hours following separation. Only feeding milk, not the physical presence of the mother, restores the heart rate. This effect is mediated by a reflex whose efferent loop is the beta-adrenergic sympathetic, cardioaccelerator nerves. Milk also regulates the peripheral resistance of young animals, which rises with an increase in alpha-adrenergic sympathetic tone in the separated rats deprived of milk (Hofer 1981).

Infant rats on separation also show a profound sleep disturbance, consisting of a delay in the onset of sleep, frequent awakenings, and a decrease in activated (rapid eye movement) sleep. The intermittent infusion of milk restores sleep to normal in separated fifteen-day-old rats.

Milk restores the metabolic rate of separated animals and assures the normal development of thermoregulation of young rats. While still poikilothermic their body temperature is also regulated by the temperature of the nest, which in turn is determined by the mother's and litter mates' body temperatures. Proper nutrition may also regulate the usual development of immune function. Levels of the catecholamine synthesizing enzymes in the adrenal medulla are reduced in weaned mice when they are separated and socially isolated (Henry et al. 1967, 1971; Axelrod et al. 1970). Separated infant monkeys rock themselves, presumably to provide their own vestibular stimulation, of which they have been deprived in the absence of a mother who rocked them while transporting them (Mason and Berkson 1974). Because separation is cited as a major stress for human beings, our understanding of its psychobiology will only be advanced by a refined analysis of its effects. Future studies will have to ask the questions: what specific facets of the interaction between two or more human beings or animals have been altered by separation, and what is the bereaved person bereft of? Is it the touch, sound, smell, sight, love, hatred, support, or income of the departed person? And how do these deprivations specifically affect the bereaved?

PSYCHOBIOLOGY OF LOSS AND SEPARATION IN ADULTS

The psychobiological correlates of separation in animals and loss in adult persons have not yet been investigated in depth or in detail. In a pioneer investigation, Wolff and colleagues (1964) studied the parents of children dying of leukemia. After an initial period of shock, disbelief, and grief on being told about their child's illness, these parents gradually came to accept it by seeking more information about it. Their sense of having caused the illness could be dispelled by a frank discussion of its nature, by information about treatment, and by advice and sympathy concerning the anticipated loss of their child.

At each stage of this proces, Wolff and colleagues accurately predicted the urinary 17-hydroxycorticosteroid (17-OHCS) levels in the parents. Their criteria for predicting these levels were the "integrity" of inferred psychological defenses (such as repression, denial, isolation, identification, etc.) and the extent of the arousal of unpleasant feelings in the parents.

These investigators also studied the characteristic differences among individual parents, with the hypothesis in mind that the more effectively a person defends himself against impending loss and its attendant feelings, the lower will be his or her mean 17-OHCS excretion rates. In twenty-three of the thirty-one instances, predictions were made from the recorded interviews of the urinary levels of 17-OHCS excretion; they supported the hypothesis that the more effective the defenses, the lower the mean 17-OHCS excretion level. Therefore, one implication of this study is that the baseline level of an individual's 17-OHCS excretion level may reflect the effectiveness of psychological defenses or other ways of coping. The same conclusion was reached for many years by many investigators (Katz 1982). However, it may not be correct in the sense that adrenal cortical excretion levels (or cortisol production and secretion) and coping strategies, although correlated, may reflect two separate and abiding characteristics of persons—not causally related.

Loss and bereavement also have significant effects on the immune system. Bartrop and co-workers (1977) studied the stimulation of phytohemagglutinin and concanavalin A, both mitogens, on the incorporation of thymidine into the lymphocytes of widows and an age-matched control population. The lymphocyte responses in the widows were lower and took six weeks to show themselves. The same result was obtained in a longitudinal study on men thirty-three to seventy-six years of age whose wives were dying of breast cancer (Schleifer et al. 1983). (Idoxuridine incorporation after mitogen stimulation was used in this study.) Significant changes were found in the spouse after the wife's death: idoxuridine incorporation was significantly lower after the first month following the spouse's demise and not before it. Recovery of function began after that and was partially completed after one year. But it is not known if this suppression of immune function is clinically meaningful—whether, for example, these men showed an increase in morbidity, infections, or malignant diseases.

Immunoglobulin levels may be affected by the stress of examinations and by maintenance or not of personal relationships. Salivary secretory immunoglobulin A levels are higher and fall less during examinations in students who maintain close, supportive ties with each other than in students who are mainly interested in grades and power. In this second group, immunoglobulin levels continued to decline even after the examination was over (Jemmott et al. 1983).

Elderly persons languishing in institutions frequently do not interact with relatives, friends, fellow inmates, or staff. The effects of such deprivation, isolation, and loss can be devastating psychologically, physiologically, and mentally. Systematic attempts at reversing this form of deprivation have now been made; they show that human contacts can be increased even in the elderly (Arnetz et al. 1983).

As the result of reversing the social isolation of some elderly persons (average age, seventy-eight years), physical and hormonal changes occurred when they were compared with similar persons who were allowed to remain by themselves. Specifically, the treated group did not lose physical stature. Estradiol and testosterone levels fell continuously in the men who remained by themselves but increased in men in the experimental group, as did plasma growth hormone levels. Dehydroisoandrosterone levels rose significantly in the first three months of increasing human contact, then fell in the socially stimulated group but continued to fall in those in whom human contact continued to remain minimal. The same trends in hormonal levels were seen in elderly women with whom social contact was maintained, but the hormonal changes were not as great in the men.

These findings are relevant to the topic of separation and isolation. They show that human relationships alter hormonal levels even in the elderly.

ONSET OF ILLNESS AND DISEASE IN THE SETTING OF LOSS

For preventive as well as for scientific reasons, the role of bereavement in disease onset should become a central concern of every medical student and physician. There are abundant observations that the health of about 67 percent of widows declines within one year of bereavement (Maddison and Viola 1968; Parkes and Brown 1972), and psychiatric morbidity increases. Parkes (1984), in a study of patients admitted to a psychiatric hospital, found that the number of patients whose illness followed the loss of a spouse was significantly greater than anticipated for people of that age and social group. Major depressions are particularly frequent in bereaved persons; in one study 45 percent became severely depressed within one year after their loss (Bornstein et al. 1973; Clayton et al. 1974). Such depressions enhance the risk of suicide and then become another (but not the only) cause for the known increases in mortality observed in survivors six months after loss (Rees and Lutkins 1967; Parkes et al. 1969; Jacobs and Ostfeld 1977).

Bereaved persons not only show a decline in health and an increase in morbidity and mortality. They also change their habits. They smoke more cigarettes and drink more alcohol—known risk factors for a variety of diseases—and use more tranquilizers (Parkes and Brown, 1972; Bornstein et al. 1973).

Less believable to many physicians is the notion that losses are the setting in which major medical diseases begin. Schmale (1958), postulating that object loss and depression are often the setting in which disease occurs, studied forty-two patients, selected for age (eighteen to forty-five years) and to some extent for social class, who were admitted to a general medical service with diagnoses ranging from hysterical conversion symptoms to aseptic meningitis. Shortly after admission each patient was interviewed using the conventional open-ended psychiatric interview. Special attention was paid to a history of loss or change in relationship with a highly valued object, and the nature of the loss was operationally divided into four categories: actual loss, threatened loss, "symbolic" loss, and no loss. In sixteen of forty-two instances, the patient either reported or the in-vestigator inferred that a loss or significant change in relationship to others had occurred within twenty-four hours of the appearance of symptoms of the disease. In another fifteen patients, such loss or change occurred within the week prior to the onset of illness. Thus thirty-one of forty-two patients experienced the onset of an illness within one week of a significant loss. Another eight patients gave a similar history for the month prior to the onset of illness. Schmale also noted that thirty-five patients experienced real or threatened loss in the first sixteen years of life. Many of these persons had unresolved conflicts with respect to these events, which were rekindled by their present illness.

A number of studies of specific diseases and the setting in which they begin have supported Schmale's observations. Real or threatened separation and bereavement have been cited as one specific factor contributing to the onset of a variety of diseases, including anorexia and bulimia nervosa (Garfinkel and Garner 1982; Strober 1984), autoimmune diseases (Paulley 1982), bronchial asthma (Rees 1964), malignancies (Kissen 1967; Bahnson 1969), diabetes mellitus (Hinkle and Wolf 1952; Stein and Charles 1971), peptic duodenal (Weiner 1977) and gastric ulcer (Peters and Richardson 1983), leukemia (Greene 1954), Graves disease (Lidz 1949), essential hyper-tension (Reiser and Ferris 1951; Weiner 1977), congestive heart failure (Perlman et al. 1971), myocardial infarction (Parkes et al. 1969), abdominal pain (Drossman 1982), ulcerative and granulomatous colitis (Engel 1955), tuberculosis (Day 1951),the complications of pregnancy and postpartum depression (O'Hara et al. 1983), and most major psychiatric illnesses (Bornstein et al. 1973). The prognosis of mycardial infarction is consider-ably worse in widowers than in age-matched married men (Chandra et al. 1983).

Young and colleagues (1963), studying mortality among widowers, found that 213 of 4,486 widowers fifty-five years old and older died within the first six months of the loss of their spouse, about 40 percent above the rate expected for married men of the same age. Kraus and Lilienfeld (1959) noted that the mortality rate of persons of both sexes who had lost a spouse was increased and that mortality was in excess of that expected in those under thirty-five years of age.

Helsing and colleagues (1981) confirmed the observations of Young and colleagues but not of Kraus and Lilienfeld. It is now quite clear that widowers are considerably more likely than married men to die between the ages of fifty-five and seventy-four years. The death of a spouse en-hances the risk of death in that age group of men especially of ischemic heart disease, for reasons and by mechanisms that we do not understand. It is likely that bereavement acts as a permissive factor in patients with coro-nary artery disease already present. Loss may play a more direct patho-genetic role in the onset of other diseases. In all these studies it is still not certain what form of grief is more likely to be correlated with disease onset. Is it the fully developed grief reaction or pathological mourning in its delayed or distorted forms?

Developing Schmale's work in the area of giving-up and its primary feelings of hopelessness and helplessness, Engel (1968) hypothesized that the "giving-up, given-up complex" is the emotional setting in which most disease occurs. He estimated that this complex precedes the onset of illness in 70 to 80 percent of patients. As with all stressful stimuli, Engel noted that it is difficult to appreciate which external stimulus will be critical to a particular person. The determining factor will be how the individual re-sponds—that is just what constitutes a loss or threatened loss will depend upon the individual's past experiences and present capacity for coping with loss. Where a serious loss is suffered or threatened, the predisposed person may react by giving-up, leading to a state of having given-up. The most characteristic feature of this process is the sense of psychological impo-tence—a feeling that for a period of time one is unable to cope with any task. Clinically, the complex is manifested by feelings of helplessness and hopelessness; low self-esteem; inability to enjoy the company of other people, one's work, hobbies, etc.; a disruption of the sense of continuity in one's past, present, and future; and a reactivation of memories of earlier periods of giving-up. Engel believes that this state of mind may last for varying periods of time and that it is commonplace for people to experi-ence this complex several times during a lifetime. In situations in which prompt resolution is impossible and periods of struggling alternate with periods of giving-up, illness may occur.

Engel's conclusions were based on his studies of patients with ulcerative colitis and on observations by Greene (1954) and Schmale (1958). Paulley (1982), however, found that pathological mourning specifically antecedes a variety of autoimmune diseases, including rheumatoid arthritis, giant cell arteritis, systemic lupus erythematosus, polymyalgia, Sjögren's syndrome, and autoimmune thyroid disease.

"CHOICE" OF DISEASE FOLLOWING BEREAVEMENT OR SEPARATION

Linear theories of disease causality would predict that an agent, stimulus, or challenge to a human being or animal would produce a specific disease. After all, streptococcus does incite erysipelas, yet it only does so if the host is also immunosuppressed. Many other factors—the dose of the infectious agent, the age of the patient, the integrity of the immune system, and bereavement—play a role in determining disease onset; a host-agent interaction must occur. Linear theories do not suffice.

Those who hold to linear, causal hypotheses of the pathogenesis of disease refute the observation that losses and bereavement are associated with the onset of a variety of diseases. Why, they ask, do such events not incite one disease alone? The answer is that neither bereavement nor streptococcus specifies a particular disease. (The streptococcus bacterium is also associated with boils, tonsillitis, rheumatic fever, acute glomerulonephritis, meningitis, and so on). The characteristics of the host determine the outcome.

Specific predispostions to a particular disease decide its nature on challenge. They specify the "choice" of the disease with which the bereaved or infected person may fall ill. They are the source of the variability of outcome. In addition, most diseases are not uniform entities. Various subforms exist whose predispositions differ.

These predispositions may be genetically determined. In the case of peptic duodenal ulcer, elevated levels of the pepsinogen I isoenzyme are a risk factor in about 60 percent of all patients with the disease; the condition is inherited as an autosomal dominant trait. The remainder of patients with duodenal ulcer have normal levels of this enzyme. Others have elevations of the pepsinogen II isoenzyme (Rotter et al. 1979).

The normotensive sons of one hypertensive parent has a more reactive cardiovascular system than one who has normotensive parents (Light 1981). In fact, many diseases run in families (Weiner 1977; Katz 1982)—a fact that is usually explained on a genetic basis. But more goes on in families than the vertical transmission of genes. In fact, intrauterine (Skolnick et al. 1980) or postnatal experiences such as premature separation (see below) place animals at risk for disease by permanently altering the levels of enzymes and disrupting rhythmic processes that regulate sleep and body temperature.

Nevertheless, the predisposition to disease takes many forms. Immunodeficiency is a risk factor for infection and for malignancies. The capacity to form immunoglobulin-E (IgE) is associated with various diseases, including atopic dermatitis, allergic rhinitis, and bronchial asthma. Yet bronchial asthma will not develop unless bronchial hyperreactivity is also present. Both these tendencies are permanent characteristics of asthmatic persons. Yet attacks of the disease are intermittent, incited by many factors including personal loss and the grief it engenders (Weiner 1977). Autoimmune factors play a role in both Graves disease and rheumatoid arthritis, yet threat (in the acute form of Graves disease) and losses (in rheumatoid arthritis) are also associated with their onset (Weiner 1977).

In one form of early essential hypertension, increased sympathetic discharge accounts for increased cardiac output, cardiac contractility, heart rate, plasma catecholamine, and renin levels but normal peripheral resistance (Julius and Esler 1975). Patients with this subform differ from other hypertension patients in their psychological makeup (Esler et al. 1975) and response to challenge (Lorimer et al. 1971). Psychological differences have also been described in two forms of rheumatoid arthritis (Rimón 1969; Vollhardt et al. 1982).

Such observations suggest that response to bereavement or separation will not be uniform. The various predispositions will determine the disease with which the person will fall ill—the "choice" of the disease. Patients with various subforms of a disease describe differences in psychological sensitivities and capacities to cope, which in turn determine their response to specific events and the way they cope with them. In other words, bereavement may play a greater role at the onset of one subform because of the specific nature of the psychobiological makeup of the host. In another subform it may play less of a determining role or none at all. The suggestion is supported by Strober (1984), who observed that anorexia nervosa patients who were characterized by binge eating experienced significantly more life stress in a six-month period than patients who remorselessly restricted their food intake or normal adolescents.

AGE AS A FACTOR IN DISEASE ONSET

The association of separation or bereavement and disease onset is in part age-dependent and in part a product of earlier experiences. However, the psychobiological responses to loss observed at a prior age in one particular system are not necessarily the same as those seen in that system at a later age. In fact, the problem of the relationship of the responses to prior experiences of separation and of responses to equivalent experiences later in the life of persons remains largely unsolved. No a priori reason exists for believing that later psychobiological responses should have the same conformation as earlier ones. One possible explanation for this discrepancy is the transformations that occur with age in every organ system. They in turn determine its response tendencies. For this reason alone bereavement may account for just a part of the pathogenetic variance in one particular age group—in enhancing, for example, the mortality of widowers age fifty-five to seventy-four.

Age-related changes have been described in at least five areas:

1. The endocrine system. The hypothalamic pituitary ovarian axis (Boyard et al. 1974) and the hypothalamic pituitary adrenal axes, with a low dehydroisoandrosterone to cortisol ratio prior to adrenarche (Rich et al. 1981), go through maturational sequences. And after menopause gonadotrophin levels rise. In anorexia nervosa, including that brought on by separation, both gonadotrophins and the adrenal hormones revert to premenarchal and preadrenarchal patterns of secretion. Amenorrhea without anorexia nervosa may also follow a young girl's leaving home— another separation.

2. The immune system. The thymus increases in size during childhood and then progressively shrinks. Eventually it fails as an endocrine organ, producing less and less thymopoeitin after age thirty to forty years, when more and more immature T-cells appear peripherally, particularly T-helper cells. Cellular immune responses are impaired. Other branches of the immune system also show age-dependent changes. Responses to a specific antigen are less vigorous. And autoantibodies—rheumatoid factors, antinuclear, and antithyroglobulin antibodies—become more prevalent. Aging is not the only variable altering immune function. Bereavement in middle age, as we have seen, also depresses T- and B-cell function, with a latent period of four to six weeks (Bartrop et al. 1977; Schleifer et al. 1983). Such a suppression also appears to occur in infants who languish in institutions. They are prone to opportunistic infections, especially viral ones, suggesting that their cellular immune system has become impaired.

Older people are prone to a variety of infections. They are at markedly increased risk for malignancies, presumably because of decreases in immune surveillance over transformed cells. Bereavement has also been cited as an onset condition for malignancy. An interaction between bereavement and impaired immune function in the elderly is, therefore, suggested.

3. The stomach. At least in rats, the main control mechanisms of gastric secretion—acetylcholine, gastrin, and histamine—go through a maturational sequence. Gastrin levels, for example, rise just before normal weaning occurs. Gastric acid secretion also goes through maturational changes. These changes may be altered by premature separation—which partly explains the finding that prematurely separated animals do not begin to develop gastric ulceration under the challenge of restraint until twenty-two days of age. Yet they are particularly prone to do so between thirty and forty days of age. Later they become decreasingly susceptible to restraint (Ackerman et al. 1975).

4. The brain. Both apical and circumferential dendrites in many areas of the brain grow and branch, then fade and eventually disappear altogether (Scheibel et al. 1977). Brain volume begins to shrink after age forty years, and cognition declines. Despite this, major behavioral manifestations of the aged brain may not occur until a separation or bereavement occurs.

5. *Circadian rhythms.* The endocrine, immune, central nervous, gastric and other systems have their own time periodicities with their own maturational sequences. To date the circadian periodic function has been studied most. Rhythmic changes occur in neurotransmitter and hormone levels, B- and T-cell function, the excretion of electrolytes and metabolites (citric acid, beta-hydroxybutyric acid and ammonia), the effects of drugs and antigens, heart rate, blood pressure, gastric secretion, temperature regulation, attention, and dreaming. But the development of these rhythmic patterns is not well known. These processes are under the control of a hierarchy of oscillators and pacemakers. The pacemakers require daily synchronization by light and personal relationships (Moore-Ede et al. 1982).

Circadian rhythms determine hours of maximal or minimal resistance to pathogenetic agents such as infection and restraint. Constraining animals at the height of their activity cycle is a potent factor in gastric ulceration (Ader 1964). The interaction of time and separation experiences at different ages is of major interest. The question of the age and timing of disease onset is complex. It can be understood in part as alterations in rhythmic time and in part as the result of disrupted personal relationships.

EXPERIMENTAL EVIDENCE THAT SEPARATION IS A RISK FACTOR
IN DISEASE ONSET

The psychobiological effects of separation on infant animals are permanent. They place these animals at risk for disease in every organ system studied to date. This generalization carries with it a provision that the factor of the age of the animal at the time of challenge must be taken into account. The results of studies on separation in animals demonstrate that it has immediate psychobiological consequences that may differ in kind from those that occur with challenges at a later age. These contentions are borne out by at least eight kinds of data:

1. *Development of high blood pressure.* Henry and colleagues (1967) studied the effects of social confrontations with members of an animal's own species and in animals with different previous experiences. They showed that mixing males from different bóxes, aggregating them in small boxes, exposing mice to a cat for many months, and producing territorial conflict in mixed males and females resulted in sustained elevations of systolic blood pressure, arteriosclerosis, and an interstitial nephritis. Higher levels of systolic blood pressure were achieved by male than by female mice who failed to reproduce under such conditions. If male mice were castrated, minimal elevations in blood presure occurred, while in those given reserpine, minimal decreases in blood pressure resulted. Earlier experiences of living together attenuated the effects on blood pressure of experimentally induced aggregation and territorial conflict. On the other hand, isolation of

animals from each other after weaning and to maturity exacerbated the effects of crowding on blood pressure levels.

Axelrod et al. (1970) and Henry et al. (1967, 1971) reported that the socially isolated male mice showed a decreased activity of tyrosine hydroxylase and phenylethanolamine N-methyl transferase activity in the adrenal gland in the baseline state. When these animals were crowded together, the effect was to increase the activity of these enzymes—an increase significantly greater than in those accustomed to crowding. The activity of both enzymes, of monamine oxidase, and the contents of noradrenaline and adrenaline in the adrenal gland were greater in these previously isolated animals who were later in constant contact with each other than in animals who were conventionally housed, i.e., crowded, but never isolated. In other words, the levels of the catecholamine synthesizing enzymes in the adrenal medulla of socially isolated male animals are lower than in animals of the same age housed together, and under social stress a marked reactive overshooting in their activity occurs.

The previously isolated male mouse becomes the dominant animal in the colony. It pays the price for its social position in the hierarchy by developing elevations of systolic blood pressure and an interstitial nephritis. Separation not only has changed the social behavior of these animals but has placed them at risk for systolic hypertension and kidney disease, from which they die.

2. *Disturbances in Pulse Rate.* Hofer and Weiner (1972, 1975) showed that a 40 percent fall in heart rate occurs (despite an increase in behavioral activity) when fifteen-day-old rats are separated from their mothers, an effect observable four hours following separation. Starting at twenty days, the heart rate of normally weaned rats falls from a level of about 420 to about 300 beats per minute. The prematurely separated animal's heart rate, having initially fallen, begins to climb and by twenty-eight days is significantly higher (350 beats per minute) than in its normally weaned peer (Hofer 1981).

3. *Disturbances in Sleep and Body Temperature Regulation.* Both in the fifteen-day-old rat and the six-month-old monkey, separation (which is followed by not eating) produces a profound sleep disturbance (Reite et al. 1974; Hofer 1976; Reite and Short 1978). Sleep onset is delayed, activated sleep is lost, rapid transitions occur between two sleep stages, sleep is fragmented, awakenings are frequent, and the animal has an overall decrease in sleep time. This sleep disturbance still occurs if the body temperature of fifteen-day-old rats is maintained within the normal range. Recovery of sleep patterns occurs by thirty days of age in these rats; they have the same sleep patterns normally weaned rats have.

When the prematurely separated animal is food-deprived or restrained at thirty days it initially falls asleep. The sleep is mainly slow-wave sleep. Such changes are not seen in normally weaned animals and are independent of changes in body temperature. Following this the prematurely separated animals show a fall in body temperature, both when food-deprived and when restrained, at which time they progressively lose sleep, mainly at the expense of slow-wave sleep (Weiner 1982).

Prematurely separated animals, therefore, respond to separation and not eating initially with one kind of sleep disturbance. At thirty days another kind of change in sleep patterns occurs when the animals are not fed, despite the fact that prior to not feeding these patterns were normal. In addition, not feeding or restraint elicits a disturbance in temperature regulation not present before challenge. These results suggest that the same challenge at two different times in the life of a separated rat produces different sleep disturbances and also elicits a disturbance in temperature regulation that had lain dormant (Ackerman et al. 1978). The fifteen-day-old rat at thirty days of age on challenge reverts to its previous poikilo-thermic state.

4. *Gastric erosions.* Prematurely separated rats when restrained or not fed (or both) at twenty-two and thirty days develop gastric erosions with an incidence of 80 to 95 percent (Ackerman et al. 1975). (The incidence in normally weaned animals is 10 percent). This effect is mediated by the aforementioned fall in body temperature (Ackerman et al. 1978). These animals do not ulcerate at seventeen days of age. After thirty days the incidence of gastric erosions declines, to become 20 percent by two hundred days of age. The effects of a challenge in prematurely separated animals is, therefore, age-related. The initial separation does not produce erosions but places animals at profound risk for lesions on subsequent challenge at a later age.

5. *Disturbances in immune function, and development of opportunistic infection.* Keller and colleagues (1983) reported that the T-cells of forty-day-old rats prematurely separated at fifteen days of age from their mothers have a significant suppression of the absolute value of thymidine incorporation into their lymphocytes after a mitogenic stimulus. The outcome of this experiment was totally unexpected: by one hundred days of age 50 percent of the prematurely separated animals (80 percent of the male and 20 percent of the female rats) had died of opportunistic—apparently viral—infections of the lungs.

6. *Disturbances in the regulation of enzyme levels.* The enzyme ornithine decarboxylase (ODC) is crucial to polyamine synthesis and therefore to growth and maturation of organs such as the heart and brain. Growth hormone is one among several regulators of ODC levels. Premature separation of rats for one hour at ten days of age lowers levels of both the hormone and the enzyme. After two hours of separation the enzyme becomes permanently unresponsive to the stimulatory effects of administered growth hormone, although it remains responsive to cycle AMP and insulin administration (Kuhn and Schanberg 1979).

7. *Growth disturbances.* Fifteen-day-old rats do not usually feed themselves during the forty-eight hours following separation. They lose weight and body temperature because they are still poikilothermic at that age.

These animals are underweight and have lowered brown body fat at thirty and forty days of age (Ackerman 1981; Keller et al. 1983). Their body weight is permanently lower than their normally weaned peers.

8. Disturbances of catecholamine and nucleoprotein content of the brain. After three days of separation the brains of fifteen-day-old pups raised at room temperature contained lower levels of catecholamines, protein, DNA and RNA. When maintained at ambient temperatures of about thirty-five degrees Celsius, the levels of norepinephrine and dopamine in the brain actually were raised but the levels of protein, DNA, and RNA continued to be depressed in the cerebrum and cerebellum, and the pups' body weights remained lower than those of their nonseparated peers (Stone et al. 1976). Whether the diminished levels of proteins and nucleoproteins continued for the duration of the lives of these animals is not known.

These observations demonstrate that separation indeed has a variety of effects that place animals at risk for disease when later exposed to social, viral, nutritional, or physical (restraint) challenges. They add substance to the belief that separation is a potent risk factor for later disease, at least in animals.

These observational and experimental data should be persuasive to students in demonstrating the crucial role of disrupted relationships in illness and disease onset. The maintenance of human relationships in stable family units is conducive to health and to buffering the effects of life stress (Cassel 1976; Cobb 1976). Supportive relationships have a therapeutic effect, for example, in reducing the number of hospitalizations of chronically ill patients. The placebo effect teaches that the mere act of being given an inert drug is therapeutic, while the proper conduct of the patient-physician relationship remains the single most powerful therapeutic tool available to medicine.

Conclusion

The argument has been made that facts about the crucial role of human relationships in health, illness, and disease can be presented in as factual a manner as any other topic. There is abundant scientific evidence of their crucial role in the maintenance of health and the onset of illness and disease. It is not necessary to appeal to or try to solicit the good will, humanity, or compassion of the student; the facts about the central role of human relationships speak for themselves. They are irrefutable and vital, not to learn them is to do a disservice to another human being—the patient.

REFERENCES

Ackerman, S. H. (1981). Premature weaning, thermoregulation and the occurrence of gastric pathology. In *Brain, Behavior and Bodily Disease* (eds. H. Weiner, M. A. Hofer, and A. J. Stunkard), 67–86. New York: Raven Press.

Ackerman, S. H., Hofer, M. A., and Weiner, H. (1975). Age at maternal separation and gastric erosion susceptibility in the rat. *Psychosomatic Medicine* 37:180–84.

Ackerman, S. H., Hofer, M. A., and Weiner, H. (1978). Early maternal separation increases gastric ulcer risk in rats by producing a latent thermoregulatory disturbance. *Science* 201:373–76.

Ader, R. (1964). Gastric erosions in the rat: Effects of immobilization at different points in the activity cycle. *Science* 145:406–7.

Arnetz, B. B., Theorell, T., Levi, L., Kallner, A., and Eneroth. P. (1983). An experimental study of social isolation of elderly people: Psychoendocrine and metabolic effects. *Psychosomatic Medicine* 45:395–406.

Axelrod, J., Mueller, R. A., Henry, J. P., and Stephens, P. M. (1970). Changes in enzymes involved in the biosynthesis and metabolism of noradrenaline and adrenaline after psychosocial stimulation. *Nature* 225:1059–60.

Bahnson, C. B. (1969). Psychophysiological complementary in malignancies: Past work and future vistas. *Annals of the New York Academy of Science* 164:319–34.

Bartrop, R. W., Luckhurst, E., Lazarus, L., Kiloh, L. G., and Perry, R. (1977). Depressed lymphocyte function after bereavement. *Lancet* 1:834–36.

Bornstein, P. E., Clayton, P. J., Halikas, J. A., Maurice, W. L., and Robins, E. (1973). The depression of widowhood after 13 months. *British Journal of Psychiatry* 122:561–66.

Bowlby, J. (1963). Pathological mourning and childhood mourning. *Journal of the American Psychanalytical Association* 11:500–41.

Boyar, R. M., Katz, J. L., Finkelstein, J. W., Kapen, S., Weiner, H., Weitzman, E. D., and Hellman, L. (1974). Anorexia nervosa: Immaturity of the 24-hour luteinizing hormone secretory pattern. *New England Journal of Medicine* 291:861–65.

Brown, J. T., and Stoudemire, G. A. (1983). Normal and pathological grief. *Journal of the American Medical Association* 250:378–82.

Butler, A. R., Suskind, M. R., and Schanberg, S. M. (1978). Maternal behavior as a regulator of polyamine biosynthesis in brain and heart of developing rat pups. *Science* 199:445–47.

Cassel, J. (1976). The contribution of the social environment to host resistance. *American Journal of Epidemiology* 104:107–22.

Chandra, V., Szklo, M., Goldberg, R., and Tonascia, J. (1983). The impact of marital status on survival after an acute myocardial infarction: A population-based study. *American Journal of Epidemiology* 117:320–25.

Clayton, P. J., Herjanic, M., Murphy, G. E., Woodruff, R., Jr. (1974). Mourning and depression: Their similarities and differences. *Canadian Journal of Psychiatry* 19:309–12.

Cobb, A. (1976). Social support as a moderator of life stress. *Psychosomatic Medicine* 38:300–14.

Day, G. (1951). The psychosomatic approach to pulmonary tuberculosis. *Lancet* 1:1025–28.

Drossman, D. A. (1982). Patients with psychogenic abdominal pain: Six years observation in the medical setting. *American Journal of Psychiatry* 139:1549–57.

Engel, G. L. (1955). Studies of ulcerative colitis: III. The nature of the psychologic processes. *American Journal of Medicine* 19:231–43.

Engel, G. L. (1968). A life setting conducive to illness: The giving-up, given-up complex. *Archives of Internal Medicine* 69:293–300.

Esler, M. D., Julius, S., Randall, O. S., Ellis, C. N., and Kashima, T. (1975). Relation of renin status to neurogenic vascular resistance in borderline hypertension. *American Journal of Cardiology* 36:708–15.

Evoniuk, G. E., Kuhn, G. M., and Schanberg, S. M. (1979). The effect of tactile stimulation on serum growth hormone and tissue orinthine decarboxylase activity during maternal deprivation in rat pups. *Communications in Psychopharmacology* 3:363–70.

Garfinkel, P. E., and Garner, D. M. (1982). *Anorexia Nervosa: A Multidimensional Perspective*. New York: Brunner/Mazel.

Greene, W. A., Jr. (1954). Psychological factors and reticulo-endothelial disease: I. Preliminary observations on a group of males with lymphomas and leukemias. *Psychosomatic Medicine* 16:220–30.

Helsing, K. J., Szklo, M., and Comstock G. W. (1981). Factors associated with mortality after widowhood. *American Journal of Public Health* 71:802–9.

Henry, J. P., Meehan, J. P., and Stephens, P. M. (1967). The use of psychosocial stimuli to induce prolonged systolic hypertension in mice. *Psychosomatic Medicine* 29:408–32.

Henry, J. P., Stephens, P. M., Axelrod, J., and Mueller, R. A. (1971). Effect of psychosocial stimulation on the enzymes involved in the biosynthesis and metabolism of noradrenaline and adrenaline. *Psychosomatic Medicine* 33:227–37.

Hinkle, L. E., Jr., & Wolf, S. (1952). A summary of experimental evidence relating life stress to diabetes mellitus. *Journal of Mount Sinai Hospital* 19:537–70.

Hofer, M. A. (1976). The organization of sleep and wakefulness after maternal separation in young rats. *Developments in Psychobiology* 9:189–206.

Hofer, M. A. (1981). Toward a developmental basis for disease predisposition: The effects of early maternal separation on brain, behavior, and cardiovascular system. In *Brain, Behavior and Bodily Disease* (eds H. Weiner, M. A. Hofer, and A. J. Stunkard). New York: Raven Press.

Hofer, M. A. (1982). On the relationship between attachment and separation processes in infancy. In *Emotion, Theory, Research, and Experience: Emotions in Early Development* (ed R. Plutchick). New York: Academic Press.

Hofer, M. A., and Weiner, H. (1972). Mechanisms for nutritional regulation of autonomic cardiac control in early development. *Psychosomatic Medicine* 34:472–73.

Hofer, M. A., and Weiner, H. (1975). Physiological mechanisms for cardiac control by nutritional intake after early maternal separation in the young rat. *Psychosomatic Medicine* 37:8–24.

Hoffman, B. (1972). *Albert Einstein: Creator and Rebel*. New York: Viking Press.

Jacobs, S., and Ostfeld, A. (1977). An epidemiological review of the mortality of bereavement. *Psychosomatic Medicine* 39:344–57.

Jemmott III, J. B., Borysenko, M., Chapman, R., Borysenko, J. Z., McClelland, D. C., Meyer, D., and Benson, H. (1983). Academic stress, power motivation, and decrease in secretion rate of salivary secretory immunoglobulin A. *Lancet* 1:1400–1402.

Julius, S., and Esler, M. D. (1975). Autonomic nervous cardiovascular regulation in borderline hypertension. *American Journal of Cardiology* 36:685–92.

Katz, J. L. (1982). Three studies in psychosomatic medicine revisited. *Psychosomatic Medicine* 44:29–42.

Keller, S. E., Ackerman, S. H., Schleifer, S. J., Schindledecker, M. A., Camerino, M. S., Hofer, M. A., Weiner, H., and Stein, M. (1983). Effect of premature weaning on lymphocyte stimulation in the rat. *Psychosomatic Medicine* 45:75.

Kissen, D. M. (1967). Psychological factors, personality, and lung cancer in men aged 55-64. *British Journal of Medical Psychology* 40:29–43.

Kraus, A. S., and Lilienfeld, A. M. (1959). Some epidemiological aspects of the high mortality in a young widowed group. *Journal of Chronic Disease* 10:207–17.

Kuhn, C. M., Butler, S. R., and Schanberg, S. M. (1978). Selective depression of serum growth hormone during maternal separation in rat pups. *Science* 201:1035–36.

Kuhn, C. M., and Schanberg, S. M. (1979). Loss of growth hormone sensitivity in brain and liver during maternal deprivation in rats. *Society of Neuroscience* (abstract) 5:168.

Lidz, T. (1949). Emotional factors in the etiology of hyperthyroidism. *Psychosomatic Medicine* 11:2–10.

Light, K. C. (1981). Cardiovascular responses to effortful coping: Implications for the role of stress in hypertension development. *Psychophysiology* 18:216–28.

Lindemann, E. (1944). Symptomatology and management of acute grief. *American Journal of Psychiatry* 101:141–48.

Lorimer, A. R., McFarlane, P. W., Provan, G., Duffy, T., and Lawrie, T. D. V. (1971). Blood pressure and catecholamine responses to stress in normotensive and hypertensive subjects. *Cardiovascular Research* 5:169–75.

Maddison, D., and Viola, A. (1968). The health of widows in the year following bereavement. *Journal of Psychosomatic Research* 12:297–306.

Mason, M. A., and Berkson, G. (1974). Effects of maternal mobility on the development of rocking and other behaviors in rhesus monkeys. *Developmental Psychobiology* 8:197–211.

Mellinkoff, S. M. (1984). Two hemispheres and the medical connection. *Pharos* 47:2–5.

Moore-Ede, M. C., Sulzman, F. M., and Fuller, C. A. (1982). *The Clocks that Time Us.* Cambridge, Mass.: Harvard University Press.

O'Hara, M. W., Rehm, L. P., and Campbell, S. B. (1983). Postpartum depression. A role for social network and life stress variables. *Journal of Nervous and Mental Disease* 171:336–41.

Parkes, C. M. (1970). The first year of bereavement. *Psychiatry* 33:444–67.

Parkes, C. M. (1971). Determination of outcome following bereavement. *Proceedings of the Royal Society of Medicine* 64:279.

Parkes, C. M. (1984). Recent bereavement as a cause of mental illness. *British Journal of Psychiatry* 110:198–204.

Parkes, C. M., Benjamin, B., and Fitzgerald, R. G. (1969). Broken heart: A statistical study of increased mortality among widowers. *British Medical Journal* 1:740–43.

Parkes, C. M., and Brown, R. J. (1972). Health after bereavement. *Psychosomatic Medicine* 34:449–61.

Paulley, J. W. (1982). Pathological mourning: A key factor in the psychopathogenesis of autoimmune disorders. Paper presented at the 14th European Congress on Psychosomatic Research.

Perlman, L. V., Ferguson, S., Bergum, K., Isenberg, E. L., and Hammarstein, J. F. (1971). Precipitation of congestive heart failure: social and emotional factors. *Annals of Internal Medicine* 75:1–7.

Peters, M. S., and Richardson, C. T. (1983). Stressful life events, acid hypersecretion and ulcer disease. *Gastroenterology* 84:114–19.

Raphael, B. (1975). The management of pathological grief. *Australia and New Zealand Journal of Psychiatry* 9:173–80.

Raphael, B. (1977). Preventive intervention with the recently bereaved. *Archives of General Psychiatry* 34:1450–54.

Rees, L. (1964). The importance of psychological, allergic and infective factors in childhood asthma. *Journal of Psychosomatic Research* 7:253–62.

Rees, W. D., and Lutkins, S. G. (1967). Mortality of bereavement. *British Medical Journal* 4:13–16.

Reiser, M. F., and Ferris, E. B. (1951). Life situations, emotions and the course of patients with arterial hypertension. *Psychosomatic Medicine* 13:133–42.

Reite, M., Kaufman, I. C., Pauley, J. D., and Stynes, A. J. (1974). Depression in infant monkeys: Physiological correlates. *Psychosomatic Medicine* 36:363–67.

Reite, M., and Short, R. (1978). Nocturnal sleep in separated monkey infants. *Archives of General Psychiatry* 35:1247–53.

Rich, B. H., Rosenfield, R. L., Lucky, A. W., Helke, J. C., and Otto, P. (1981). Adrenarche: Changing adrenal response to adrenocorticotropin. *Journal of Clinical Endocrinology and Metabolism* 52:1129–35.

Rimón, R. (1969). A psychosomatic approach to rheumatoid arthritis. *Acta Rheumatica Scandinavia* 13 (suppl. I).

Rotter, J. I., Sones, J. Q., Samloff, I. M., Richardson, C. T., Gursky, J. M., Walsh, J. H., and Rimoin, D. L. (1979). Duodenal-ulcer disease associated with elevated serum pepsinogin I: An inherited autosomal dominant disorder. *New England Journal of Medicine* 300:63–66.

Scheibel, M. E., Tomiyasu, U., and Scheibel, A. B. (1977). The aging human Betz cell. *Experimental Neurology* 56:598–609.

Schleifer, S. J., Keller, S. E., Camarino, M., Thornton, J. C., and Stein, M. (1983). Suppression of lymphocyte stimulation following bereavement. *Journal of the American Medical Association* 250:374–77.

Schmale. A. H., Jr. (1958). Relation of separation and depression to disease I: A report on a hospitalized medical population. *Psychosomatic Medicine* 20:259–77.

Skolnick, N. J., Ackerman, S. H., Hofer, M. A., and Weiner, H. (1980). Vertical transmission of acquired ulcer susceptibility in the rat. *Science* 208:1161–63.

Stein, S. P., and Charles, E. (1971). Emotional factors in juvenile diabetes mellitus: A study of early life experience and adolescent diabetics. *American Journal of Psychiatry* 128:700–704.

Stone, E., Bonnet, K., and Hofer, M. A. (1976). Survival and development of maternally deprived rats: Role of body temperature. *Psychosomatic Medicine* 38:242–49.

Strober, M. (1984). Stressful life events associated with bulimia in anorexia nervosa: Empirical findings and theoretical speculations. *International Journal of Eating Disorders* 3:3–16.

Vollhardt, B. R., Ackerman, S. H., Grayzel, A. I., and Barland, P. (1982). Psychologically distinguishable groups of rheumatoid arthritis patients: A controlled, single blind study. *Psychosomatic Medicine* 44:353–62.

Weiner, H. (1977). *Psychobiology and Human Disease.* New York: Elsevier.

Weiner, H. (1982). The prospects for psychosomatic medicine: Selected topics. *Psychosomatic Medicine* 44:488–517.

Wolff, C. T., Friedman, S. B., Hofer, M. A., and Mason, J. W. (1964). Relationship between psychological defenses and mean urinary 17-hydroxycorticosteroid excretion rates. *Psychosomatic Medicine* 26:576–91.

Young, M., Benjamin, B., and Wallis, C. (1963). The mortality of widowers. *Lancet* 2:454–56.

T W O

Symptoms without Signs

Somatic Presentation of Psychiatric Illness

GEOFFREY G. LLOYD

In all clinical specialties doctors are consulted by patients whose somatic symptoms are not supported by the diagnosis of any significant somatic pathology. A substantial proportion of these patients suffer from various types of psychiatric illness, and from the viewpoints of diagnosis and management, they pose some of the most difficult problems in clinical medicine. Indeed, there have been claims that this is an area where doctors fail to do justice to their patients' symptoms so that emotional problems are overlooked and unnecessary physical investigations are instigated. Some doctors appear more likely than others to miss or ignore emotional cues, concentrating only on the presenting somatic complaints and thereby reinforcing the patient's conviction that he is physically ill. Sensitivity and interviewing style are crucial if the doctor is to identify the psychological disorder beneath the somatic facade, and fortunately these are skills that can be improved with appropriate tuition. This is therefore a major topic for medical education during medical school and postgraduate training.

This presentation of illness has recently become known as somatization, a term that has been defined in various ways but which has three essential components. First, the patient presents with somatic symptoms for which no organic basis can be found. Second, the symptoms are attributed by the patient to organic disease, this attribution often persisting long after reassurance has been given that physical examination and investigations have been negative. Third, specific questioning reveals an underlying psychological disorder that can account for the presenting somatic complaints. The frequency with which this occurs clinically is becoming increasingly recognized, but somatization has a long history extending back over several centuries. Indeed, its ubiquity is such that it should perhaps be regarded as a basic mechanism for manifesting distress. The presentation of emotional distress with psychological symptoms ("psychologization") appears to be the

24

more recent phenomenon and is still uncommon in many cultures (Goldberg and Bridges 1988).

One of the earliest systematic studies was conducted by Cabot (1907) at Massachusetts General Hospital in Boston. He examined the case notes of all patients attending the outpatient department of this prestigious hospital and found that nearly half had no organic disease to account for their symptoms. He described these patients as having functional disease, and some of the diagnoses assigned to them at the time now make interesting historical reading. They include neurasthenia, gastroptosis, cardiac neurosis, and uterine misplacements. The term functional disease has now been discredited, and we tend to look for positive evidence of psychiatric illness in this group of patients. Several recent studies have used standardized measures of assessment, confirming the high prevalence of psychiatric morbidity without organic pathology in patients attending various medical facilities (Lloyd 1983).

One of the most influential studies was that carried out in primary care by Goldberg and Blackwell (1970). Using a standardized clinical interview, they found that 30 percent of patients attending a family doctor's surgery had evidence of various types of psychiatric morbidity, but one-third of them were not recognized by their doctor and were only detected by a research psychiatrist using a standardized interview. Patients in this group, who have been described as constituting the hidden psychiatric morbidity of general practice, were not recognized as such because they formulated their illnesses, to themselves and to their doctors, almost exclusively in physical terms. It is almost certainly from this group that patients are refered by their doctors to various hospital departments according to the nature of their symptoms, thus explaining why so many clinics contain patients with no organic pathology.

A more recent study in primary care has suggested that somatization is even commoner than previously believed (Bridges and Goldberg 1985). Over half the patients in this study presenting to their general practitioners with a new episode of psychiatric illness satisfied criteria for somatization. Thirty-two percent presented entirely with somatization. Another 24 percent were categorized as facultative somatizers in that they did not attribute their somatic symptoms to physical illness when interviewed by a research psychiatrist although they had done so when they consulted their general practitioner. Only 17 percent presented with psychological symptoms of their psychiatric disorder. The majority of somatizing patients remain under their general practitioner's care with frequent excursions to hospital specialists. Psychiatrists had little contact with such patients until the recent widespread establishment of liaison services in general hospitals and psychiatric clinics in primary care. However, even when a psychological explanation for their symptoms is suspected these patients often resist psychological exploration, refuse psychiatric referral, and demand a further round of physical investigations.

Presenting Symptoms

Psychiatric illness can present with a wide range of symptoms localized to almost any part of the body, but certain symptoms predominate and their pattern can often give a strong indicator as to the true nature of the patient's problems. Pain is one of the most common symptoms in this group of patients. Previous generations of students were taught to think of pain as indicating tissue damage, but we now know that in many cases pain is largely psychogenic in origin; in other words, it can be best understood in a psychological rather than a somatic framework. Bond (1978) described the characteristic features of psychogenic pain. Its onset is poorly defined, it is decribed in vague terms, it does not conform to anatomical distributions of dermatomes or peripheral nerves, it may be relieved by alcohol, psychotropic drugs, or nothing at all. Psychogenic pain can occur in almost any part of the body, but some sites are particularly frequent, especially the head, chest, and abdomen. When pain is a manifestation of a depressive illness it may dominate the clinical picture to such an extent that the patient does not appear depressed; a depressed mood and the other cognitive aspects of depression may only be admitted after specific questioning. Psychiatrists and clinical psychologists now make a significant therapeutic contribution in pain clinics, specifically established for the management of patients with chronic pain. In many of these patients psychological factors greatly outweigh physical factors in etiology, either through a specific psychiatric illness or because of abnormal illness behavior.

Headache and facial pain are common symptoms of psychiatric illness seen at neurological clinics. Facial pain can also be a presenting symptom to dentists and oral surgeons, and it has been shown quite clearly that pain of this nature responds well to treatment with tricyclic antidepressants (Feinmann et al. 1984). Other neurological symptoms include dizziness, special sensory disturbance, and impairment of high intellectual functions such as concentration and memory. Motor paralysis is a recognized manifestation of hysteria, the incidence of which appears to be declining. Other hysterical phenomena include gait disturbances, pseudoseizures, and sensory loss. Neurological examination usually allows these symptoms to be distinguished from those due to organic disease. For example, weakness of a limb can be shown to be associated with simultaneous contraction of agonistic and antagonistic muscles. During examination, there is discontinuous resistance, wasting is absent, and reflexes are normal.

Cardiologists encounter psychiatric illness presenting with chest pain. There is a long history describing the evolution of theories of nonorganic chest pain, and several of the clinical reports have come from military medicine. One of the best known was provided by Da Costa (1871) on the basis of his observations during the American Civil War. He described soldiers who were invalided from battle because of chest pain, palpitations, breathlessness, dizziness, and abnormal fatigability. He belived that this syndrome, which was subsequently known for some time as Da Costa's syndrome, was the result of abnormal innervation of the heart. Later, during the First World War, Thomas Lewis (1920) coined the term *effort syndrome*. From his observations during the Second World War, Paul Wood (1941) advocated that this term be dropped because "a proper psychiatric diagnosis is nearly always possible." He believed that the fundamental feature was the establishment of a link between the emotional reaction and effort, this link coming about through a variety of mechanisms, including misinterpretation of emotional symptoms, a conviction that the heart was to blame, and a consequent fear of sudden death on exertion. Recent work has shown that patients with chest pain who are investigated for cardiac disease but who prove to have no significant coronary obstruction have higher levels of psychiatric morbidity than those who do have coronary artery disease (Bass and Wade 1984). Anxiety neurosis was the commonest diagnosis; the patients had a wide range of phobic and anxiety symptoms, especially a fear of crowds and of being in enclosed spaces.

Respiratory difficulties are closely associated with cardiac symptoms. There are many reports of sighing respiration in patients suffering from the effort syndrome, and in the 1930s hyperventilation was considered to be responsible for all the symptoms of this syndrome, being due to an underlying anxiety state. Patients attending general medicine or respiratory medicine clinics may therefore have symptoms without pulmonary disease or symptoms that are disproportionately severe in relation to pulmonary disease. Respiratory disorders of psychological origin are essentially abnormalities of the rate and rhythm of breathing due to a persistent faulty habit or to a psychiatric illness that promotes episodic hyperventilation. The accompanying biochemical changes may themselves cause symptoms that overshadow both the respiratory complaint and psychiatric illness. In extreme form hypocapnia produces tetany and loss of consciousness; in milder cases it causes dizziness, fatigue, palpitations, chest pain, and paraesthesiae.

Prominent gastrointestinal symptoms include anorexia, weight loss, vomiting, abdominal pain, and bowel disturbance. At least a fifth of a series of gastrointestinal outpatients were shown to have a psychiatric illness without organic disease (MacDonald and Bouchier 1980). Some patterns of gut symptoms have attracted particular interest. Persistent vomiting is one such example, either in isolation or as part of a syndrome of anorexia nervosa or bulimia nervosa. The irritable bowel syndrome has also been studied from a psychiatric viewpoint. The characteristic features of this condition are abdominal pain that is relieved by defecation, abdominal distension, and frequent loose stools at the onset of pain. These features occur in the absence of organic disease of the gut. Controlled studies have shown a higher prevalence of psychiatric morbidity among patients attending hospital clinics, although the relationship between abdominal and psychological symptoms has not been fully explained (Creed and Guthrie 1987). In some patients psychological symptoms of an anxiety state or depressive illness have clearly antedated the bowel complaints and may well have had an etiological role in the development of the irritable bowel syndrome. When the bowel symptoms are chronic the development of a psychiatric illness or stressful life events may lower the patient's tolerance and lead him or her to seek medical referral.

Family doctors and gastroenterologists are seeing increasing numbers of patients with vague symptoms of ill health which they attribute to food allergy. Pearson et al. (1983) assessed twenty-three patients with complaints of allergies to food and found evidence for hypersensitivity in only four patients, all of whom had other features of atopy. The patients without allergy had high levels of neurotic symptoms, similar to those seen in a psychiatric outpatient population (Rix et al. 1984). The authors concluded that symptoms attributed to food allergy actually had a psychogenic basis, but the patients were hostile to this explanation and persisted in viewing their illness as organic, with the result that they confined themselves to dangerously restricted diets.

Gynecologists are often consulted by patients with pelvic pain, vaginal discharge, and menstrual irregularities for which no organic pathology can be found. These symptoms have been shown to be especially prevalent around the time of menopause (Gath et al. 1987). Menorrhagia without objective evidence of disease has been shown to be associated with psychiatric morbidity (Greenberg 1983). It has also been demonstrated in women undergoing hysterectomy for benign menorrhagia that levels of psychiatric morbidity were higher than in the general population but fell significantly postoperatively (Gath et al. 1982). Therefore it seemed likely that psychosocial factors were important influences on referral and selection for surgery. Younger women may present with infertility or sexual problems and complete amenorrhoea may lead the girl with anorexia nervosa to consult a gynecologist. Other genital symptoms arouse the suspicion of venereal disease: pain in the penis, pruritis ani, and offensive smells from the genitalia. Up to 30 percent of patients attending a genitourinary clinic have no objective evidence of infection, and we are now seeing patients who have neurotic fears of having contracted AIDS without any laboratory evidence that they actually have done so.

The belief that one is infected may be held with delusional intensity. Dermatologists are consulted by patients delusionally convinced that they are infested with skin parasites. This symptom may be part of a widespread psychiatric disorder such as schizophrenia or depressive psychosis, but in some cases there is no other psychopathology and the delusion remains unchanged for years. Classification of this symptom is controversial, but some authorities regard it as a monosymptomatic hypochondriacal psychosis.

Dermatitis artefacta is another unusual condition that masks psychiatric disorder. The patient presents with necrotic, ulcerating lesions with a sharp, geometrical outline; these lesions are seldom distributed symmetrically but occur in sites accessible to the patient's dominant hand. They are chronic and recur despite repeated treatment. Although the lesions are self-inflicted the patient does not admit to this until several consultations have taken place; even then in some cases the artifactual nature of the condition is strongly denied. Many kinds of psychiatric illnesses, personality problems, and social difficulties are associated with this symptom, and recovery is often determined more by personality maturation and improved life circumstances than by medical treatment (Sneddon and Sneddon 1975).

Attention has been drawn to the disturbance of body image that accompanies skin complaints, usually associated with depression (Cotterill 1981). The most striking disorder of body image is the generalized disturbance associated with anorexia nervosa, but localized disorders lead to specific requests for cosmetic surgery. The patient complains of ugliness or deformity in one part of the body, which to any observer appears quite normal or only minimally disfigured. The nose, chin, ears, and breasts are the most common sources of complaint in this condition, to which the term *dysmorphophobia* has been applied. Some follow-up studies have shown that patients with minor deformities may derive considerable benefit from surgery, but a recent report has described a high rate of neurosis and schizophrenia with patients who had had a rhinoplasty for cosmetic reasons rather than for disease or trauma (Connolly and Gipson 1978). Psychological and social background should therefore be considered carefully before surgery is undertaken, and a specialized psychiatric opinion should be sought in difficult cases.

Underlying Psychiatric Syndromes

Although psychiatric illness is common among patients with medically unexplained symptoms, some patients do not warrant a psychiatric diagnosis. They may be reacting temporarily to stressful life events and can be expected to improve physically once this stress is resolved. Alternatively they may, by nature, be sensitive to normal bodily sensations without experiencing any major disruption to their lives. In other cases no explanation, either physical or psychological, can be found after thorough assessment; sometimes the true nature of the condition is revealed only by long-term follow-up (Lloyd 1983).

When psychiatric illness is diagnosed it has been difficult to classify according to any established nosology. However, this task has been made easier by the introduction of DSM III. In this context an especially important development has been the inclusion of a separate group of somatoform disorders. The essential features of these disorders are physical symptoms suggesting physical disorders for which there are no demonstrable organic findings or known physiological mechanisms; there also has to be evidence that the symptoms are linked to psychological factors or conflicts. This group has displaced the category of hysterical neurosis by splitting it into a number of categories defined in terms of their presenting symptoms. These categories are somatization disorder, conversion disorder, psychogenic pain, hypochondriasis, and atypical somatoform disorder. Somatization disorder is almost synonymous with the condition formerly known as Briquet's syndrome. Its cardinal features are multiple, recurrent somatic complaints occurring in many parts of the body and starting before age thirty. It is almost exclusively confined to women, and its prevalence appears to be higher in the United States than in the United Kingdom, perhaps because Americans have easy access to specialists of all types and thus might more readily develop the multiple complaints on which the diagnosis is based (Lloyd 1986a). Conversion disorder is characterized by loss or distortion of neurological function which cannot be fully explained by neurological disease. Psychogenic pain, a new distinct diagnostic category, is defined as pain that is not associated with any physical condition, does not conform to a recognized anatomical distribution, and for which psychological factors are regarded as paramount in onset or maintenance. The essential feature of hypochondriasis is an unrealistic and morbid interpretation of bodily sensations leading to the fear or belief of having serious disease. The preoccupation with disease, which persists despite negative investigations and medical reassurance, causes major impairment in social functioning. Hypochondriasis in this context is not secondary to any other psychiatric disorder such as depressive illness or anxiety state. The other category of atypical somatoform disorder is used for those conditions in which there is preoccupation with a perceived defect in physical appearance for which cosmetic surgery is demanded; this is sometimes known as dysmorphophobia.

The creation of new diagnostic categories is not entirely convincing. The somatoform syndromes merge with one another and also with the factitious disorders, such as dermatitis artefacta and Munchausen's syndrome, in which symptoms are initiated voluntarily by the patient (Lloyd 1986b). The distinction between somatoform and factitious disorders depends on the judgment of whether symptoms are produced consciously or unconsciously. This is a subjective judgment notoriously difficult to make and is further complicated if the patient's insight varies from time to time, which often appears to be the case.

Among patients referred to hospital clinics with medically unexplained symptoms, somatoform disorders are likely to predominate when the symptoms are chronic. In the majority of patients with symptoms of recent onset, depressive illness and anxiety disorders are the more common diagnoses. If the correct diagnosis is to be made, it is esential that the interview be conducted in such a way as to encourge the patient to describe his or her mood, current concerns, and personal background. Psychological problems do not form part of the presenting complaints of somatizing patients and may even be denied at first on direct questioning if the patient is overwhelmingly fixated on physical disease. By skilled probing, however, an experienced interviewer will be able to uncover changes of mood and the other cognitive aspects of depression or anxiety.

Why Do Patients Somatize?

It has already been pointed out that somatization is a much older phenomenon than psychologization and can be regarded as a basic human reaction to stress. Indeed, it is such an ingrained aspect of behavior that it may carry certain advantages; these will be discussed later, but first let us consider some of the reasons why it occurs.

People who somatize may perceive normal bodily sensations as more intense and more unpleasant than do people who do not somatize. Furthermore, they interpret these sensations in a morbid way, attributing them to physical pathology and thus believing themselves to be seriously ill. Once this pattern of thinking is established it tends to be perpetuated because all subsequent sensations are interpreted in such a way as to reinforce the preoccupation with sickness. It has been proposed that some people are unable to express their feelings verbally because of a neurophysiological deficit that prevents them experiencing fantasy and affect (Barsky and Klerman 1983). This phenomenon, often called alexithymia (Nemiah 1977), is thought to be associated with a tendency to focus on the details of external events and an inability to express inner drives. It may well be one of the psychological characteristics of somatizing patients.

A further explanation of somatizing behavior is derived from the concepts of the sick role, illness behavior, and learning theory. Thus it is considered that the behavior is adopted because of the rewards that the sick role conveys, namely the attraction of sympathy and care and the avoidance of unacceptable responsibilities. The pattern of behavior may have been learned initially by modeling on someone else who derived secondary gain from illness or by direct personal experience based on previous episodes of illness. This explanation explains why some somatizing patients respond so poorly to treatment. The advantages of the sick role, as far as these patients are concerned, outweigh the benefits of cure, so they respond badly to any intervention that seeks to remove them from the sick role. Barsky and Klerman (1983), who reviewed these explanations in detail, proposed that an "amplifying somatic style" is the most suitable concept for describing the underlying disposition to present distress in terms of somatic symptoms. This is free of clinical assumptions and etiological theories. The patient with an amplifying somatic style may or may not have a diagnosable psychiatric disorder, mood disturbance, emotional conflict, or associated physical illness.

Whatever the basic psychological characteristic, there is little doubt that somatization is greatly influenced by social and cultural factors. It is commoner among the elderly and lower socioeconomic groups; it may also be influenced by a family history or previous personal history of physical illness. There is consistent agreement that it is much more common in people from developing countries than it is in Western cultures. Perhaps the greater stigma attached to psychiatric illness in these countries is a factor that helps shape the presentation of symptoms to a doctor. However, there is also evidence that the native languages in many developing countries do not have a rich vocabulary of emotional expression. Words to describe depression or anxiety may simply not exist, so it is almost inevitable that emotional distress has to be expressed through somatic complaints (Leff 1981).

It is from a cultural perspective that the advantages of somatization can be understood best. Some of the advantages have been summarized by Goldberg and Bridges (1988). First, somatization allows people for whom psychiatric illness is unacceptable or who live in a culture that stigmatizes psychiatric illness nevertheless to occupy the sick role when psychologically unwell. Second, it enables them to avoid blame or responsibility for their illness. Third, it appears to protect them from feeling as depressed as they might otherwise. These advantages apply to a lesser extent in Western cultures where psychiatric illness is relatively more acceptable. They then have to be set against the disadvantages, among which are included the morbidity of hazardous and inappropriate investigations and the failure to receive the correct treatment for a reversible condition.

Management

One reason why these patients prove so difficult to manage is that their perception of the nature of their illness differs markedly from that of their doctor. Optimum management depends crucially on the correct diagnosis being made as quickly as possible after presentation. This can prevent the establishment of a pattern of abnormal illness behavior, which is notoriously difficult to alter once it has become chronic. A detailed history should be taken of the presenting complaints so that they can be fully evaluated; it is also important that the patient feels his symptoms are not being dismissed lightly. Psychological symptoms should be inquired about, with particular emphasis on any temporal relationship between emotions, life stress, and the presenting somatic complaints. A family and personal history should be taken. Physical examination must be carried out by the doctor whom the patient consults initially, focusing on that part of the body which is the site of symptoms. Appropriate investigations should be requested and completed as quickly as possible. It can often be useful to request a specific investigation even if it is expected to be normal; this enables the patient to be reassured and strengthens the doctor's evidence against organic pathology. Referral to specialists should be made sparingly and after careful consideration. However, once a psychological diagnosis is made physical examination and investigations should stop unless there are new and unexpected symptoms. Clinical management is probably more likely to be successful if the doctor can alter the patient's attribution of his symptoms from organic to psychological. The negative physical examination and laboratory results should be summarized and discussed. Reasons for concluding that the symptoms are psychological should be explained, together with a description of the somatic symptoms of the relevant psychiatric disorder, for example, anxiety or depression. It can be revealing to ask whether the patient has ever observed an association between somatic symptoms and emotions in relatives or friends. Prognosis is best when somatization has an acute onset and short duration at the time of presentation. A depressive illness or anxiety disorder can often be diagnosed, in which case there is a good response to conventional treatment with antidepressant drugs or behavior therapy. Management is more difficult when symptoms are due to a chronic disorder such as hypochondriasis, psychogenic pain, or somatization disorder. Some patients with these disorders are among the least insightful and least cognitively oriented encountered in medical practice, so psychodynamic therapy is unlikely to be beneficial (Murphy 1982). Nevertheless, clinical impression suggests that the doctor-patient relationship can be used therapeutically if the physician is prepared to establish a long-term empathic relationship (Monson and Smith 1983). The patient should be seen regularly by the same physician so that he or she does not have to produce new symptoms to see a doctor. A regular relationship will also discourage inappropriate multiple consultations with different specialists. Whether the patient is managed by a family doctor or psychiatrist is of lesser importance than the consistency of the relationship. Psychiatrists are becoming more experienced in treating these patients, but many patients are stubbornly resistant to psychiatric referral; management therefore has to remain in the hands of the family doctor. The symptoms should be understood as a method of emotional communication and related to problems in the patient's personal life. Psychotropic drugs have little part to play except in cases where there are definite affective symptoms. Improvement may only occur following changes in social circumstances, and the doctor should do what he can to foster social change, always being prepared to accept that his role is more likely to be supportive than curative.

REFERENCES

Barsky, A. J., and Klerman, G. L. (1983). Overview: Hypochondriasis, bodily complaints and somatic styles. *American Journal of Psychiatry* 140:273–83.
Bass, C., and Wade, C. (1984). Chest pain with normal coronary arteries; a comparative study of psychiatric and social morbidity. *Psychological Medicine* 14:51–61.

Bond, M. R. (1978). Psychological and psychiatric aspects of pain. *Anaesthesia* 33:355–61.

Bridges, K. W., and Goldberg, D. P. (1985). Somatic presentation of DSM III psychiatric disorders in primary care. *Journal of Psychosomatic Research* 29:563–69.

Cabot, R. C. (1907). Suggestions for reorganization of hospital outpatient departments with special reference to improvement of treatment. *Maryland State Medical Journal* 50:81–91.

Connolly, F. M., and Gipson, M. (1978) Dysmorphophobia: A long-term study. *British Journal of Psychiatry* 132:568–70.

Cotterill, J. A. (1981). Dermatological non-disease: A common and potentially fatal disturbance of cutaneous body image. *British Journal of Dermatology* 104:611–19.

Creed, F., and Guthrie, E. (1987). Psychological factors in the irritable bowel syndrome. *Gut* 28:1307–18.

Da Costa, J. M. (1871). On irritable heart: A clinical study of a functional cardiac disorder and its consequences. *American Journal of Medical Science* 61:17–52.

Feinmann, C., Harris, M., and Cawley, R. (1984). Psychogenic facial pain: presentation and treatment. *British Medical Journal* 288:436–38.

Gath, D., Cooper, P., and Day, A. (1982). Hysterectomy and psychiatric disorder: I. Levels of psychiatric morbidity before and after hysterectomy. *British Journal of Psychiatry* 140:335–42.

Gath, D., Osborn, M., Bungay, G., Iles, S., Day, A., Bond, A., and Passingham, C. (1987). Psychiatric disorder and gynaecological symptoms in middle aged women: A community survey. *British Medical Journal* 294:213–18.

Goldberg, D. P., and Blackwell, B. (1970), Psychiatric illness in general practice: A detailed study using a new method of case identification. *British Medical Journal* 2:439–43.

Goldberg, D. P., and Bridges, K. (1988). Somatic presentation of psychiatric illness in primary care setting. *Journal of Psychosomatic Research* 32:137–44.

Greenberg, M. (1983). The meaning of menorrhagia: An investigation into the association between the complaint of menorrhagia and depression. *Journal of Psychosomatic Research* 2:209–14.

Leff, J. P. (1981). *Psychiatry around the Globe: A Transcultural View.* New York: Dekker.

Lewis, T. (1920). *The Soldier's Heart and the Effort Syndrome.* London: Shaw.

Lloyd, G. (1983) Medicine without signs. *British Medical Journal* 287:539–42.

Lloyd, G. G. (1986a). Hysteria: A case for conservation? *British Medical Journal* 293:1255–56.

Lloyd, G. G. (1986b). Psychiatric syndromes with a somatic presentation. *Journal of Psychosomatic Research* 30:113–20.

Macdonald, A. J., and Bouchier, I. A. D. (1980). Non-organic gastrointestinal illness: A medical and psychiatric study. *British Journal of Psychiatry* 136:276–83.

Monson, R. A., and Smith, G. R. (1983). Current concepts in psychiatry: Somatization disorder in primary care. *New England Journal of Medicine* 308:1464–65.

Murphy, G. E. (1982). The clinical management of hysteria. *Journal of the American Medical Association* 247:259–64.

Nemiah, I. C. (1977). Alexithymia. *Psychotherapy and Psychosomatic* 28:199–206.

Pearson, D. J., Rix, K. J. B., and Bentley, S. J. (1983). Food allergy: How much in the mind? An objective clinical and psychiatric study of suspected food hypersensitivity. *Lancet* 1:1259–60.

Rix, K. J. B., Pearson, D. J., and Bentley, S. J. (1984). A psychiatric study of patients with supposed food allergy. *British Journal of Psychiatry* 145:121–26.

Sneddon, I., and Sneddon, J. (1975). Self-inflicted injury: A follow-up study of 43 patients. *British Medical Journal* 3:527–30.

THREE

███████

Psychiatry in Medicine

Cost-Effectiveness Studies

JAMES J. STRAIN, GEORGE FULOP, JEFFREY S.
HAMMER, AND JOHN S. LYONS

Emily Mumford and Herbert Schlesinger began a new genre of critical studies to assess the relationship between medical illness and the utilization of mental health services (Mumford et al. 1978, 1982, 1984; Schlesinger 1980, 1983). In their pioneering research, they began to focus not only on the issue of costs of mental health care but ingeniously upon the intimate relationship between the consumption of mental health and general health resources. Until their efforts, this interface of mental and physical comorbidity and costs had been a no man's land for scientific inquiry, except for anecdotal statements and commentaries. More specifically, Mumford and Schlesinger highlighted the intimate relationship between mental health treatment and medical care utilization in a fee-for-service system. Their research addressed exactly how the provision of mental health services diminishes the costs of general medical care and for whom. These studies were seminal for several reasons:

1. Mental health care had always been underfunded, and in even greater danger of attrition in the era of cost-containment that is heralded by the skyrocketing costs of medical care in the 1970s and 1980s.

2. Although noncompliance—a behavioral phenomenon—has long been recognized as one of the most important problems in medicine, the role of other behaviors and mental disorders per se upon the use of general medicine service was poorly understood.

3. The necessary concepts, constructs, and confounds that underlie the scientific examination of medical and psychiatric comorbidity had heretofore been inadequately specified.

4. The reliability and validity of the instruments used to evaluate mental disorders or the severity of medical illness were markedly compromised. Both the interaction of the physical symptomatology on mental phe-

35

nomena and the impairment of physical functioning by mental factors severely confounded analyses.

There is little doubt that the cutting edge investigations of Mumford and Schlesinger set in motion a flurry of excitement and interest in the cost-offset effects of a psychosocial intervention with regard to (1) enhancement of the patient's mental well-being, (2) diminution of unnecessary medical examinations and hospitalizations, and (3) important policy considerations for third-party reimbursement for mental health services. Further testimony to the debt that we owe Mumford and Schlesinger is evidenced by the establishment of the American Psychiatric Association Task Force on Cost-Effectiveness of Consultation/Liaison Psychiatry, the emphasis on the promotion of cost-offset studies by the National Institute of Mental Health (NIMH), including its pioneering workshops to generate fundable grant initiatives from potential investigators, and the eventual NIMH support of at least ten ongoing research efforts. Our great regret is that Emily Mumford could not tell her own story.

Nevertheless, this chapter will attempt to describe the epidemiological evidence for the important relationship between mental disorders and primary medical care, the definitions of the various constructs for cost-offset and cost-effectiveness, the early evidence of the cost-offset benefits from mental health care delivery on the ultimate costs for total health care, strategies for the design and construction of cost-offset studies, results from a preliminary NIMH-funded study, and policy implications for the future of research and the funding of mental health services.

Background: Mental Health and General Medical Care

As the principal gatekeeper for much of the mental health care system, primary care physicians (PCPs) inevitably encounter and, thus, need to assess, triage, manage, refer, and treat vast numbers of people with alcoholism, drug abuse, and mental disorders. With regard to PCPs in this role, Pincus and Kamerow, in a report to the Administrator of Alcohol Drug Abuse Mental Health Administration (ADAMHA), not only describe overwhelming evidence of their importance, but question the effectiveness of treatment.

And the role of the PCP takes on added significance when it is realized that 62% of persons with mental disorders are seen exclusively in the general medical setting. The Epidemiological Catchment Area (ECA) study reports that 19% of American adults in any 6-month period experience anxiety (8.3%), affective disorders (6%), and alcohol (5%) and drug abuse (2%) problems (Regier et al. 1984). In 1983, alcoholism, drug abuse, and mental disorders (ADM) resulted in at least 108,000 deaths per year: 69,000 alcohol-related (up to one-half of all motor vehicle crash deaths involve alcohol), 6,000 associated with drug abuse, and 33,000 mental health-related, primarily suicides (Hoeper et al. 1979a).

The cost of these disorders further underscores their importance. In 1983, ADM disorders resulted in 50.4 billion dollars in direct and 250 billion dollars in indirect costs (HCFA 1984). More than half of all hospitalized patients manifest significant psychologic dysfunction, either as a result of, or in conjunction with, medical illness that can interfere with the effectiveness of treatment; furthermore, between 15% and 50% of all patients encountered in the ambulatory medical setting have psychologic dysfunction that is either primary in nature or secondary to physical illness (Lipowski 1967a).

Regier et al. (1984) estimate that only 21% of this group receives care from mental health specialists. Although 70% of patients with an ADM disorder (in the previous 6 months) made at least one ambulatory health or mental health visit, only 10% saw a mental health specialist (Shapiro et al. 1984). Even though more than half of those with ADM disorders received all their care in the general medical sector (usually from a primary care physician), only one-fifth stated that they made a visit for mental health purposes. In developing countries, the World Health Organization has declared that the provision of mental health care is by necessity via the PCP and physician extenders (International Conference 1978).

However, these data do not consider the quality of care patients with ADM disorders receive, especially in view of the fact that despite their high prevalence rates they frequently go undetected by the PCPs. In one study, 2.8% were recognized by the physicians as opposed to 27% that were diagnosed by the research team (Hoeper et al. 1979b). This extremely low recognition rate has added significance because the figure included *any* indication of recognition, e.g., chart notation or a psychotropic drug prescription. Only 25% to 50% of patients with major depression were identified by PCPs (Schulberg et al. 1985; Nieson and Williams 1980). Significant undetected cognitive disturbances were observed by Knight and Folstein (1977), as well as by Jacobs et al. (1977). Of the estimated 10% of all adults entering a physician's office who are likely to have a problem with alcohol, relatively few are detected. Despite this problem in recognition and diagnosis, Unlenhuth et al. (1980) found that 70% of tricyclic antidepressants (TCAs) and 90% of anxiolytics are administered by PCPs.

With regard to treatment, surveys show that despite the high proportion of TCA use by PCPs, there is an inappropriately low rate of antidepressant and high rate of antianxiety medications prescribed for their patients with major depression (Unlenhuth et al. 1980). Admittedly, the tricyclic antidepressants are useful for certain types of depression, but they are commonly prescribed in subtherapeutic doses by PCPs. Furthermore, referral rates to a mental health clinician for a recognized mental disorder are disturbingly low (Shepherd et al. 1966; Thompson et al. 1983; Cohen-Cole et al. 1982). Even less treatment and referral information is available for drug and alcohol disorders seen in primary care. However, physicians commonly restrict their attention to the medical complications of alcohol rather than to the disease itself (Jones and Helrich 1972), and they remain pessimistic about their abilities to effectively treat the disorder (Weschler et al. 1983). Only 5% of the PCPs surveyed report that they were "very successful" in helping their patients with drug and alcohol use problems (Jones and Helrich 1972).

There are many barriers to improving the mental health care provided by PCPs: the PCPs' inadequate training, knowledge, and negative attitudes toward their delivery of mental health care (Weschler et al. 1983; Strain et al. 1983; Shine and Demas 1984); patients' denial of their psychological problems and their negative attitudes about seeking mental health care and/or accepting referral; constraints within the health care systems, e.g., cost; availability of psychiatrists; and the lack of integrated medical and mental health service systems (Pincus 1980). These barriers overlap and interact to decrease the likelihood of effective mental health care for patients seen in primary care settings.

With regard to inpatients, Fulop et al. (1987) documented the impact of psychiatric comorbidity on the medical and surgical patients' hospital course, including their length of stay (LOS), in two university teaching hospitals. The discharge abstracts of all medical and surgical patients hospitalized in 1984 at the Mount Sinai Hospital in New York City (N = 37,370) and from Northwestern Memorial Hospital in Chicago (N = 21,889) were reviewed. Only those patients whose principal diagnoses were medical or surgical were included. Patients on the medical/psychiatric units were excluded. The data at Mount Sinai Hospital were collected on the Utilization Information Services hospital discharge abstract form (Utilization Information Services 1983). This data base includes length of stay, demographic data, and diagnoses—an admitting diagnosis, a retrospectively determined principal diagnosis for the condition that resulted in the admission, and up to six secondary diagnoses. The psychiatric diagnoses on the abstracts were made by psychiatric consultants (18%) and primary physicians (82%). The data at Northwestern Memorial Hospital were obtained from the hospital discharge summary abstract and included only demographic data, diagnoses, and length of stay.

All inpatients were divided according to the presence or absence of a psychiatric comorbidity. Psychiatric comorbidity was defined as any ICD-9-CM/DSM-III psychiatric diagnosis (codes 290–319) in any secondary diagnostic entry. The average LOS and geometric mean LOS were derived for both groups. (The geometric mean LOS represents the central tendency for a distribution of whole number integers. Given that number of days in the hospital meets this criterion, the geometric mean may be a less biased estimate of the population central tendency and also serves to decrease the skewedness of the geometric distribution [Hays 1981].)

The patients with psychiatric comorbidity in both Mount Sinai Hospital and the Northwestern Memorial Hospital stayed significantly longer (table 1). The geometric mean LOS was also greater for the patients with psychi-

Table 1. Length of Stay for All Medical/Surgical Patients and for Medicare Beneficiaries with and without Psychiatric Comorbidity at Two Hospitals

Group	Number of Patients	Length of Stay (Days)				Comparison of Length of Stay[b]		
		Mean	SD	Range	Geometric Mean[a]	t	df	p
All medical/surgical inpatients								
Mount Sinai Hospital								
Psychiatric comorbidity	2,009	19.8	33.3	1–791	10.7	14.1	37,368	.0001[c]
No psychiatric comorbidity	35,361	9.2	15.3	1–738	5.4			
Northwestern Memorial Hospital								
Psychiatric comorbidity	811	13.7	27.7	1–88	8.7	10.8	21,887	.0001[c]
No psychiatric comorbidity	21,078	8.3	13.2	1–43	5.2			
Medicare beneficiaries								
Mount Sinai Hospital								
Psychiatric comorbidity	969	24.3	33.6	1–508	14.1	9.1	10,028	.0001[c]
No psychiatric comorbidity	9,061	14.2	20.0	1–529	8.3			
Northwestern Memorial Hospital								
Psychiatric comorbidity	416	15.3	26.8	1–87	10.1	6.9	8,009	.001[c]
No psychiatric comorbidity	7,595	10.4	12.8	1–45	6.9			

[a] The geometric mean reduces skewing of the sample distribution and may be a less biased estimator of central tendency.
[b] Significance assessed with two-tailed t test assuming unequal subsample variance.
[c] Significant at overall .05 level (Bonferroni procedure p value of <.0125).

Source: Fulop et al., *Am J Psychiatry* 144:879. Copyright 1987, The American Psychiatric Association. Reprinted by permission.

atric comorbidity. These patients were significantly older, less likely to be female, and more likely to be black or Hispanic. Examination of the admission, hospital course, and discharge characteristics revealed that significantly more of the medical/surgical patients with psychiatric comorbidity had been admitted in emergency situations (49.0% versus 23.0%; $X^2 = 725$, df = 1, p<.001) and from other health care facilities (5.8% versus 1.1%; $X^2 = 339$, df = 1, p<.001). Their hospital courses were characterized by significantly more consultations (mean ± SD = 1.4 ± 1.6 versus 0.5 ± 1.0; t = 26.3, df = 37,368, p<.001), operative procedures (mean ± SD = 2.4 ± 1.8 versus 2.0 ± 1.5; t = 11.1, df = 37,368, p<.001), and medical diagnoses (mean ± SD = 3.8 ± 1.7 versus 3.0 ± 1.8; t = 21.1, df = 37,368, p<.0001). Finally, the medical/surgical patients with psychiatric comorbidity were significantly more likely to die (8.0% versus 3.3%; $X^2 = 125$, df = 1, p<.0001) or to be discharged to a long-term care facility (10.5% versus 1.5%; $X^2 = 774$, df = 1, p<.001).

Fulop et al. also described eight ICD-9/DSM-III categories and the associated length of stay of the medical/surgical inpatients (table 2). The organic mental disorders accounted for 27.1% of the psychiatric diagnoses and were predominantly substance-induced or secondary to physiologic processes and not dementias arising in the senium and presenium. Substance use and affective disorders were also prevalent.

The overall rates of psychiatric consultation among all patients and those with Medicare insurance were 1.9% (N = 697) and 3.2% (N = 317), respectively. Among the outliers (patients whose hospital stays were greater than two standard deviations above the Medicare mean length of stay), 8.5% (N = 305) received psychiatric consultations.

Since a greater mean LOS and geometric mean LOS were found for patients with psychiatric comorbidity on general hospital wards at two different university hospitals, the results are unlikely to be an idiosyncratic characteristic of either site. Within several DRG categories, the presence of a psychiatric diagnosis was associated with a longer mean LOS. This extended hospital stay among patients with psychiatric comorbidity may be secondary to more severe medical illnesses, the additional diagnostic and treatment time required by the psychiatric disorders, or psychopathology that confounds the treatment and management of the medical disorders.

However, it is essential to exercise caution in the interpretation of the study findings. First, whereas estimates of psychiatric comorbidity in medical/surgical inpatients range up to 30%–50% (Lipowski 1967b), the rate of detection of psychiatric disorders in this study was only 5%. Second, even though an independent study of the abstraction process found a low rate of diagnosis coding errors (Data Quality Assessment Report 1986), the reliability and validity of the nonpsychiatrist's descriptions and the medical record abstractor's coding of the psychiatric disorders remain an issue. Although only 18% of the patients receiving psychiatric diagnoses had psychiatric consultations, this is similar to the 11.5% rate found in a national

Table 2. Psychiatric Diagnoses and Associated Length of Stay for 2,009 Medical/Surgical Inpatients with Psychiatric Comorbidity at Mount Sinai Hospital

Psychiatric Disorder[a]	Patients with Diagnosis[b]		Length of Stay (Days)			
	N	%	Mean	SD	Range	Geometric Mean
Organic mental disorder						
DSM-III section 1						
Dementia	39	1.9	29.7	41.3	1–173	14.8
Substance-induced organic mental disorder	132	6.6	17.3	35.4	1–366	8.5
DSM-III section 2 —organic mental disorder secondary to physiologic process	483	24.0	23.6	33.4	1–508	14.5
Substance use	561	30.5	13.1	17.3	1–264	7.6
Affective disorder	366	18.2	26.9	33.6	1–273	15.2
Other disorder	193	9.6	18.2	59.5	1–791	7.6
Psychosis	180	9.0	23.3	33.0	1–314	13.5
Anxiety	146	7.3	14.5	15.7	1–88	8.6
Adjustment disorder	75	3.7	27.8	27.7	1–172	17.6
Personality disorder	61	3.0	16.4	23.0	1–150	9.2

[a] Determined by ICD-9/DSM-III codes.

[b] Each patient may have had more than one DSM-III category of psychiatric diagnoses. The 2,009 medical/surgical patients with psychiatric comorbidity had a mean±SD of 1.2±0.5 psychiatric diagnoses.

Source: Fulop et al., *Am J Psychiatry* 144:880. Copyright 1987, The American Psychiatric Association. Reprinted by permission.

probability sample of all patients in short-term general hospitals (Wallen et al. 1987).

Third, the difference between the groups with and without psychiatric comorbidity in admission, hospital course, and discharge variables were not covaried in the current analysis. These variables would be suitable control variables in prospective hypothesis-testing studies. Fourth, the notably higher rate of psychiatric consultation among the outliers suggests an alternative hypothesis: the longer one stays in the hospital, the more likely it is that a psychiatric disorder will manifest itself, be detected, or engender negative feelings in physicians that lead them to call for a psychiatric consultation. This may increase the rate of diagnosis of psychiatric disorders among longer-stay patients. An intriguing clinical question remains: why did the patients with psychiatric diagnoses appear more ill, i.e., have significantly more emergency admissions, consultations, and operative procedures, and have a greater likelihood of dying or being discharged to long-term care facilities?

Definitions of Cost-Effectiveness in Medicine

A major difficulty confronting the strategies and tactics for either the study, the design, or the interpretation of cost-effectiveness studies in general and for mental health service delivery within the medical setting in particular is the selection of the appropriate construct for assessing and defining costs (Doubilet et al. 1986; Ludbrook 1986; Fahs 1986; Moloney and Rogers 1979; Angell 1985; Schwartz 1987; Marcus 1987).

Doubilet et al. (1986) provide a scholarly and comprehensive review of the various approaches to defining cost constructs and provide a conceptual framework for assessing their value and utility depending upon the question that is being asked and the availability of explicit data. For example, some of the more common uses of the term *cost-effective* include (1) cost saving, (2) only effectiveness, (3) cost savings with an equal (or better) health outcome, or (4) having an additional benefit worth the additional costs. To illustrate the confusion that results when different definitions are applied, the authors examine the utility of strategies that evaluate Papalonicolou smears in screening for cervical cancer: "According to criterion 1, it is not cost-effective to screen at all, since to do so would involve a net expenditure of money. According to criterion 2, on the other hand, it is not only cost-effective to screen, but increasing the screening frequency increases cost-effectiveness. Criterion 3 does not allow the comparison of screening strategies on the basis of cost-effectiveness [in the data provided]. . . . Finally, when criterion 4 is applied, whether or not screening is determined to be cost-effective depends on the amount of money one is willing to pay for each additional year of life." The authors suggest that the term *cost-effective* should be restricted to cases where criterion 4 applies.

When criterion 1 or 2 is employed, the term *cost-effective* should be avoided and the construct of "cost savings" or "most effective" employed.

However, it is important to note that many medical decisions cannot be made on the basis of costs alone, and that the psychological meaning of the treatment (e.g., the reassurance of a negative test) may outweigh the monetary cost-effectiveness and is an integral part of good, as well as ethical, medical practice. Similarly, the savings from the cost reduction in the length of hospital stay should be balanced by the patient's psychological need (especially if living alone) to have another day of hospitalization for recuperation and rehabilitation to better withstand a long convalescence at home.

Intervention Studies: Mental Health Treatment and Reduced Cost of Medical Utilization

As early as 1941, Billings (1941) observed that the average LOS was 28 days among patients with psychiatric comorbidity but only 15 days when such patients received a timely psychiatric diagnosis and subsequent involvement of the psychiatric liaison service. In a study of discharge abstracts from short-term general hospitals with and without psychiatric units between 1970 and 1977, patients with psychiatric disorders diagnosed according to the hospital adaptation of ICDA (H-ICDA-2 1973) stayed an average of 10.8 days, whereas the mean stay of all patients (including the patients with psychiatric comorbidity) was 7.3 days (Wallen 1985).

Mumford et al. (1984) reviewed the outcome of twenty studies examining the impact of a psychosocial intervention. In a West German investigation in 1963, Duehrssen and Jorswiek (1965) reported that the cost of outpatient psychotherapy may be offset by savings in medical expenditures. Specifically, those patients who had psychoanalysis or psychoanalytic psychotherapy had a decreased use of hospitalization during a 5-year observation period in comparison to a control group. Jones and Vischi (1979) report that psychotherapy could reduce the utilization of medical services by 20%. In a study of coronary patients, where LOS was included as an outcome variable, "psychologically treated" patients were discharged 2 days earlier than an untreated group (Mumford et al. 1982). Finally, a meta-analysis of 49 controlled experiments on the effect of psychoeducational interventions with surgical patients revealed 1.31 fewer hospital days than for the control group (Devine and Cook 1983).

Mumford et al. (1984) again examined 58 controlled studies using meta-analysis, and identified the variables associated with decreased use of medical resources following mental health intervention. In the same study, Mumford and her coworkers had access to the Blue Cross and Blue Shield Federal Employees Program, a large and independent data set which allowed them to reexamine the same hypotheses from different points of view to overcome idiosyncratic results and the lack of generalizability.

By analyzing only those 22 studies that were not biased by patient's self-selection or subject to the phenomenon of "regression to the mean," Mumford et al. learned that the modest psychological interventions employed in these studies were associated with a reduction in inpatient hospital days, specifically, 1.5 below the nonintervention group's average stay of 8.7 days. In another group of nonrandomized studies (N = 26), which were naturalistic studies of patients who had selected psychotherapy for themselves, a 33% reduction in the utilization of medical resources followed the use of mental health services. Furthermore, both the meta-analysis and Blue Cross/Blue Shield claims database studies revealed that the cost-offset effect was more likely to be greater for inpatients than outpatients and that older patients had greater offset effects than younger patients following mental health treatment. Such offset findings were not consistently observed in outpatient settings where mental health treatment users also had higher medical costs.

It is important to note that Mumford et al. suggest a reduced rate of *increase* of medical expenses follows mental health treatment. Since 75% of total medical charges are accounted for by inpatient charges, enhanced maintenance of health status and reduction of inpatient costs as a result of timely mental health care would have profound effects. Furthermore, "since evidence shows that those receiving mental health care suffer more chronic disease and are physically sicker than those who do not use psychiatric services, the effects of outpatient mental health treatment cannot be explained as simple substitution of one outpatient service for another." Appropriately used psychiatric service would free misused medical services for those who really need it.

Two key psychiatric intervention studies that followed the Mumford et al. observations were those conducted by Smith et al. (1986a) and Levitan and Kornfeld (1981). Smith et al. (1986b) reviewed the literature that reported that patients with multiple physical symptoms but no apparent physical disease (somatization disorder) use up to 9 times the average per capita amount of medical care. Employing a randomized, controlled study design, Smith et al. observed that in comparison with the control group, those receiving a psychiatric consultation had a decrease in quarterly health charges of 53% ($p \geq 0.05$). In the cross-over phase of their study, once the control group received an intervention there was also a reduction in quarterly health charges of 49%. The authors formulated that psychiatric consultation for patients with somatization disorder reduced health care costs, and this effect was not related to changes in health status or the patients' satisfaction with their health care.

In a seminal study, Levitan and Kornfeld demonstrated that following a psychiatric liaison intervention, elderly women (65 years of age or older) who were admitted for an emergency surgical repair of a fractured femur experienced a significant reduction in hospital LOS: 30 versus 42 days in the control group, and a greater likelihood to return home than go to a nursing home. For a $10,000 investment in a psychiatric liaison intervention that effectively screened and treated all patients in the experimental year (in contrast to the rarely referred patient for psychiatric consultation in the control year), $192,000 in hospital and posthospital cost savings were estimated.

This investigation also highlights the importance of the screening method—liaison psychiatry in the medical/surgical setting—where all high-risk patients are screened and treated for mental health needs, in contrast to the traditional psychiatric consultation model that only allows for evaluation of those few patients referred to psychiatry, who often have gross and the most severe manifestations of behavioral abnormalities (Strain and Grossman 1975). A prospective investigation of these two psychiatric intervention methods and their outcome are described below.

Finally, the need for a timely screening intervention has been demonstrated by Lyons et al. (1986), who documented that the earlier inpatients are seen in psychiatric consultation, the more likely they are to remain in hospital for a shorter length of time. Specifically, Lyons et al. derived a timing variable calculated using the following formula:

$$\text{Timing} = \log \frac{(days\ prior\ to\ consult)}{\log (LOS)}$$

Since LOS and days prior to consult were both positively skewed, logarithmic transformations were applied to both. The mean LOS for the sample studied was 22.0 days and the median LOS was 13.8 days. The mean number of days the patient stayed in the hospital prior to psychiatric consultation was 8.2 days and the median was 4.3 days.

A simple linear regression model was used to predict the transformed LOS variable using the "Timing variable." The Pearson correlation coefficient between these two variables was 0.342 ($p<0.001$). The following regression equation was obtained:

$$y = 0.447x + 0.874,$$

where y is the log (LOS) and x is the Timing variable defined above (figure). The strong positive relationship between these two variables indicates that the sooner the consult, the shorter the length of stay. The timing of the psychiatric consultation, as measured presently, accounted for nearly 12% of the variation of LOS for these patients.

To help ensure that this effect was not due to some difference in the type of patient who received early versus late consultation, patients who received consultation in the first half of their hospital stay were compared with patients receiving consultation in the second half (table 3). There were

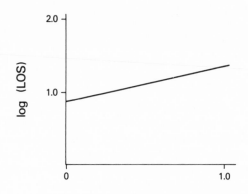

Timing of Psychiatric Consultation

Regression line demonstrating the relationship between the timing of psychiatric consultation and hospital length of stay.

no significant differences between early and late consultation patients with regard to medical versus surgical and with regard to the most frequently occurring psychiatric diagnoses.

By suggesting that early consultation may be more cost-effective than late consultation, the results also offer indirect support for the notion that psychiatric consultations can reduce the costs of a patient's general hospital care. In the Lyons study, the average proportion of stay prior to consultation was 0.52. If, on the average, this timing could be reduced to 0.40, the present model would predict an approximately 1.5-day reduction in average length of stay. Across the 419 patients studied, this would mean a cost savings of at least $250,000, based on reduced bed days. In addition, the timing methodology employed may serve as a useful model for a more refined study of the efficacy of the consultation process. For instance, the slope of this regression line can be compared across DRGs or across psychiatric diagnoses and other patient characteristics to determine differential efficacy across these dimensions.

Research Design Considerations

Studies done to date are compromised by several design confounds that plague the study of psychiatric disorders and their treatment in the medically ill. For example, in most studies, no attempt was made to specify the psychosocial services provided the control (nonintervention) patients. Therefore, the control groups were contaminated, at least in part, by unspecified psychosocial interventions. Levitan and Kornfeld used the patients on the same unit prior to the liaison intervention as their "control" group (Strain 1981). Consequently, other factors could explain the results (e.g., staffing or attending physician changes, policy shifts, alterations in medical/surgical procedures, case mix differences, etc.). Since the distribution of LOS is almost always skewed to the right, mean differences may be misleading without proper data transformations (e.g., logarithmic). Other methodological problems include: (1) lack of randomized sampling techniques, (2) inadequately defined inclusion criteria, (3) use of psychological measures without established reliability and validity, (4) raters not blind to the hypotheses or the nature of the intervention, (5) inadequate observation periods, (6) no specification of severity of disease state or utilization of valid instruments for its assessment, (7) lack of specification of psychosocial disability, (8) insufficient delineation of the intervention or measurement of its intensity, (9) sample sizes too small to accurately estimate population parameters, and (10) a limited range of cost metrics. Berk (personal communication) also argues persuasively for the need to consider both direct and indirect costs and to address the question of costs to whom—government, third-party payers, patients, or patients' families. The study reported below, conducted by Strain, Hammer, Lyons, Fahs, Strauss, Lebovits, Paddison, and Snyder, was designed to overcome the confounds presented by the studies reported to date.

The Cost-Offset Effects from a Prospective Study

Strain et al. (1988), funded by an NIMH grant, conducted a prospective study to examine the cost-offset effects of a psychiatric liaison intervention with elderly patients. The subjects were consecutively admitted patients to

Table 3. Percentages of Early and Late Consultations by Medical versus Surgical and Psychiatric Diagnoses

Patient Type	% Early	% Late
Medical	90.4	87.9
Surgical	9.6	12.1
DSM-III Diagnosis		
Adjustment disorders	15.1	14.4
Organic brain syndromes	14.1	10.3
Dysthymic disorder	12.1	13.2
Alcohol/drug abuse	5.5	4.6
Personality disorders	4.0	5.2
Schizophrenia	4.0	2.9
Anxiety disorders	2.0	2.9
Major affective disorders	1.5	1.7
Other/deferred/missing	31.7	34.8

Source: Lyons et al., *Gen Hosp Psychiatry* 8:161. Copyright 1986 by Elsevier Science Publishing Co., Inc. Reprinted by permission.

three orthopedic wards (two units at Northwestern Memorial Hospital [NMH] and one unit at Mount Sinai Hospital [MSH], NYC) 65 years or older for a surgical repair of a fractured hip. Several instruments were employed: a semistructured interview, a chart-review inpatient log, the Beck Depression Inventory, the Arthritis Impact Measurement Scale, the Spielberger State-Trait Anxiety Inventory, the Horn Disease Staging Evaluation, and the Research Diagnostic Criteria. Each patient was interviewed at admission and discharge and at 6 weeks and 12 weeks postdischarge.

The first 12-month period was a baseline on all three units. During the second year, a liaison psychiatry intervention was introduced at Mount Sinai and on one of the Northwestern units and consisted of the following: (1) every consenting patient was evaluated by a psychiatrist and offered treatment if necessary; (2) weekly ombudsman rounds with a senior orthopedic attending (Strain and Hamerman 1978); (3) weekly nursing and discharge planning meetings; and (4) conferences with families and social workers as appropriate.

The authors report that at MSH, the consultation rate was 10% (N = 12) in the control year and 80% (N = 115) in the intervention or screen year. In the screen year, 20% would not consent or died during the hospitalization. Fifty-six percent of the intervention year patients at MSH had the diagnosis of an organic mental disorder (OMD) and this percentage was significantly higher than that of the general consultation cohort (p≤.0001). In contrast to the control cohort, the intervention patients (N = 115) stayed in the hospital 2.0 days less at $600/day for a savings of $172,500. The NWM intervention cohort were in hospital for one day less ($600 per day), decreasing hospital costs by $22,848. The psychiatrists made 282 patient visits to the MSH intervention cohort, which could have generated $21,760 in fees ($80/visit) to offset the psychiatrist's salary of $20,000 to perform the consultations. There was no difference in discharge placement for the control compared to the intervention cohort.

Public Policy Implications

The association between longer LOS and psychiatric comorbidity has implications for public policy and patient care. For instance, although each diagnosis related group (DRG) was designed to represent a homogeneous group of inpatients who make "equal" use of hospital resources, considerable variability within DRGs has been observed; the relative insensitivity of DRGs to issues complicating individual cases (e.g., comorbidity or severity of illness) has also been documented (Horn et al. 1985; Berki et al. 1984).

The current DRG reimbursement mechanism provides incentives for treatment plans that are focused but not generalized or comprehensive, thereby creating a disincentive for measures aimed at the primary or secondary detection of psychiatric comorbidity in the medically ill. Even though many psychiatric disorders experienced during medical hospitalizations are transient (Sensky 1985), once detected the mental disorders are undertreated and unlikely to receive appropriate psychiatric treatment after hospitalization (Karasu et al. 1977; Burstein 1984). Furthermore, the lack of detection of psychiatric disorders not only endangers psychiatric aftercare but also threatens compliance with the prescribed medical regimen (Stam and Strain 1985; Strain 1978).

If it is discerned that psychiatric detection and intervention result in savings, then strategies for fiscal incentives for the identification and treatment of psychiatric disorders should be undertaken through the DRG system. Perhaps the transfer of select patients with psychiatric comorbidity to psychiatric-medical units not regulated by DRGs would promote the treatment of psychiatric disorders discovered on medical units (Fogel et al. 1985). This would facilitate appropriate psychiatric disposition and protect against the undertreatment of psychiatric morbidity. Premature hospital discharge of patients with psychiatric comorbidity because of the LOS constraints imposed by DRG fiscal incentives may also be prevented.

However, specialized treatment units, as well as all psychiatric units, may soon lose their prospective payment system exemption, removing this fiscal option. In fact, Fogel et al. reported that under DRGs, specialized medical/psychiatric units (primarily medical) fared worse financially than the DRG-exempt psychiatric/medical units (primarily psychiatric). Unless special considerations for psychiatric comorbidity are included in a new DRG reimbursement formula, treatment of patients with psychiatric comorbidity will likely result in deficits for hospitals.

Conclusion

Additional studies are essential to more adequately understand mental health treatment and its effects on medical utilization. These studies need to incorporate the important dilemmas that confound the results obtained to date, (e.g., case mix, measurement of severity of physical illness, assessment of mental disorders in the medically/surgically ill, the development of adequate and pragmatic cost models, and the application of micro- and macro-economic assessment strategies for direct and indirect costs). Necessary future studies include: (1) cross-sectional epidemiological surveys of psychiatric comorbidity in the hospitalized medically/surgically ill; (2) prospective studies examining all medical/surgical inpatients at admission and discharge for the presence of psychiatric disorders and determining the associated LOS; (3) multivariate model building to assess the effect of independent variables (e.g., psychiatric comorbidity, psychosocial characteristics, demography, and severity of medical and psychiatric illness) on LOS; (4) studies of the cost effectiveness of psychosocial intervention with regard to LOS; and (5) the effect of DRGs on the detection and/or treatment of psychiatric comorbidity. Such studies may elucidate the mechanism underlying the role of psychiatric comorbidity and costs and have major policy implications for early identification and treatment of psychiatric comorbidity in the medical setting.

Without a doubt, the data in this chapter indicate the debt we owe to Emily Mumford and her coworkers for their pioneering studies involving the cost offsets that accrue from timely psychiatric interventions in the medical setting. Their efforts set in motion a new generation of studies that have important health care and policy implications. If future studies continue to replicate that for targeted groups (the elderly) in specific settings (the inpatient surgical setting), psychiatric treatment not only improves patient care but reduces the utilization of medical resources as well, then (in the words of Scharfstein and Beigel 1984) patients can have "more for less."

The consideration of cost issues in the practice of medicine is essential for the education of tomorrow's physician. Just as Engel has so clearly articulated the need for biological, psychological, and social components to be incorporated into the clinical decision-making process, it is clear from the foregoing that physician evaluation of cost parameters should be an essential ingredient in the clinical decision-making process. Furthermore, in the education of the doctor, it is important that the tools be provided to speak for the patient on the policy level as well: allocation of scarce resources; governmental support of medical care for catastrophic illness (e.g., HIV, cardiac transplantation, etc.); provision of mental health coverage from third-party payers; and participation in the decision-making process to diminish medical expenses when the expected benefit to the patient is minimal (e.g., procedures undertaken solely to avoid malpractice vulnerability). The need to understand the issues of costs in medicine is a core competence in the education of the physician for his/her optimal care of the patient.

ACKNOWLEDGMENTS

We would like to thank Susan M. Sonenreich for her editorial assistance. This research has been supported by NIMH grant MH40790 and the Green Fund.

REFERENCES

Angell M: Cost containment and the physician. *JAMA* 254:1203–1207, 1985.
Berk A: Overview of cost studies of hospitalization. (In draft form, personal communication to JJ Strain).
Berki SE, Ashcraft ML, Newbrander WC: Length-of-stay variations within ICDA-8 diagnosis-related groups. *Med Care* 22:126–142, 1984.
Billings EG: Value of psychiatry to the general hospital. *Hospitals* 15:305–310, 1941.
Burstein A: Psychiatric consultations in a general hospital: Compliance with follow-up. *Gen Hosp Psychiatry* 6:139–141, 1984.

Cohen-Cole SA, Bird J, Freeman A, et al.: An oral examination of the psychiatric knowledge of medical house staff: Assessment of needs and evaluation baseline. *Gen Hosp Psychiatry* 4:103, 1982.

Data Quality Assessment Report, Albany, NY Hospital Association of New York State, 1986.

Devine EL, Cook TD: A meta-analytic analysis of effects of psychoeducational interventions on length of postsurgical hospital stay. *Nurs Res* 3:267–274, 1983.

Doubilet P, Weinstein MC, McNeil BJ: Use and misuse of the term "cost effective" in medicine. *New Engl J Med* 314(4):253–256, 1986.

Duehrssen A, Jorswiek E: An empirical and statistical inquiry into the therapeutic potential of sychoanalytic treatment. *Der Nerenarzt* 37:166–169, 1965.

Fahs MC: Letter to the editor re: Use of the term "cost effective." *New Engl J Med* 314:1645, 1986.

Fogel BS, Stoudsmire A, Houpt JL: Contrasting models for combined medical and psychiatric inpatient treatment. *Am J Psychiatry* 142:1085–1089, 1985.

Fulop G, Strain JJ, Vita J, Lyons JS, Hammer JS: Impact of psychiatric comorbidity on length of hospital stay for medical/surgical patients: A preliminary report. *Am J Psychiatry* 144:828–833, 1987.

Hays W: *Statistics,* 3d ed. New York, Holt, Rinehart & Winston, 1981.

Health Care Financing Administration 1983 Figures. Quoted in *Washington Post,* October 17, 1984.

Hospital Adaptation of ICDA, 2d ed. (H-ICDA-2). Ann Arbor, Michigan, Commission on Professional and Hospital Activities, 1973.

Hoeper EW, Nycz GR, Cleary PD, Regier DA, Goldberg ID: Estimated prevalence of RDC mental disorder in primary medical care. *Int J Ment Health* 8:6–15, 1979a.

Hoeper EW, Mycz G, Cleary PD: The quality of mental health services in an organized primary health care setting. Final report, NIMH Contract No. 278-79-0013 (DB), 1979b.

Horn SD, Bulkley G, Sharkey PD, et al.: Interhospital differences in severity of illness: Problems for prospective payment based on diagnosis-related groups (DRGs). *N Engl J Med* 313:20–24, 1985.

International Conference on Primary Health Care, WHO and UNICEF, Alma Ata, Russia, September 1978.

Jacobs J, Bernhard MR, Delgado A, Strain JJ: Screening for organic mental syndrome in the medically ill. *Ann Intern Med* 86:40–46, 1977.

Jones KR, Vischi TR: Impact of alchohol, drug abuse and mental health treatment on medical care utilization. *Med Care* 17 (Dec. suppl.), 1979.

Jones RW, Helrich AR: Treatment of alchoholism by physicians in private practice. *Q J Stud Alcohol* 33:117–131, 1972.

Karasu RB, Plutchik R, Steinmuller RI, et al.: Patterns of psychiatric consultation in a general hospital. *Hosp Community Psychiatry* 28:343–347, 1977.

Knights EB, Folstein MF: Unsuspected emotional cognitive disturbances in medical patients. *Ann Intern Med* 87:723–728, 1977.

Levitan SJ, Kornfeld DS: Clinical and cost benefits of liaison psychiatry. *Am J Psychiatry* 138:790–793, 1981.

Lipowski ZJ: Review of consultation psychiatry and psychosomatic medicine I and II. *Psychosom Med* 29:153–171, 201–224, 1967a.

Lipowski ZJ: Review of consultation psychiatry and psychosomatic medicine, II: Clinical aspects. *Psychosom Med* 29:201–224, 1967b.

Ludbrook A: Letter to the editor re: Use of the term "cost effective." *New Engl J Med* 314:1645, 1986.

Lyons JS, Hammer JS, Strain JJ, Fulop G: The timing of psychiatric consultation in the general hospital and length of hospital stay. *Gen Hosp Psychiatry* 8:159–162, 1986.

Marcus DD: Cost containment: How is it to be achieved? *JAMA* 257:228, 1987.

Moloney TW, Rogers DE: Medical technology: A different view of the contentious debate over costs. *New Engl J Med* 301:1413–1419, 1979.

Mumford E, Schlesinger HJ, Glass GV: A critical review and indexed bibliography of the literature up to 1978 on the effects of psychotherapy on medical utilization. Report to NIMH. Contract NIMH-MH-77-0049. Rockville, MD, NIMH, 1978.

Mumford E, Schlesinger HJ, Glass GV: The effects of psychological intervention on recovery from surgery and heart attacks: An analysis of the literature. *Am J Public Health* 72:141–151, 1982.

Mumford E, Schlesinger HJ, Glass GV, Patrick C, Cuerdon T: A new look at evidence about reduced cost of medical utilization following mental health treatment. *Am J Psychiatry* 141:1145–1158, 1984.

Nieson AC, Williams TA: Depression in ambulatory medical patients: Prevalence by self-report questionnaire and recognition by nonpsychiatric physicians. *Arch Gen Psychiatry* 37:999–1004, 1980.

Pincus HA: Linking general health and mental health systems of care: Conceptual models of implementation. *J Psychiatry* 137:315–320, 1980.

Pincus H, Kamerow D: Personal communication.

Regier DA, Myers JK, Kramer M, Robins LN, Blazer DG, Hough RL, Eaton WW, Locke BZ: The NIMH Epidemiologic Catchment Area (ECA) Program: Historical context, major objectives, and study population characteristics. *Arch Gen Psychiatry* 41:934–941, 1984.

Scharfstein SS, Beigel A: Less is more? Today's economics and its challenge to psychiatry. *Am J Psychiatry* 141:1403–1408, 1984.

Schlesinger HJ, Mumford E, Glass GV: Mental health services and medical utilization. In: Vandenbos G (ed.), *Psychotherapy: From Practice to Research to Policy.* Beverly Hills, CA, Sage Publications, 1980.

Schlesinger HJ, Mumford E, Glass GV, et al.: Mental health treatment and medical care utilization in a fee-for-service system: Outpatient mental health treatment following the onset of a chronic disease. *Am J Public Health* 73:422–429, 1983.

Schulberg HC, Saul M, McClelland M, et al.: Assessing depression in primary medical and psychiatric practice. *Arch Gen Psychiatry* 42:1164–1170, 1985.

Schwartz WB: The inevitable failure of current cost-containment strategies: Why they can provide only temporary relief. *JAMA* 257:220–224, 1987.

Sensky T: Failure to keep psychiatric follow-up appointments (letter). *Gen Hosp Psychiatry* 7:272–273, 1985.

Shapiro S, Skinner EA, Kessler LG, Von Korf M, German PS, Tischler GL, Leaf PJ, Benham L, Cottler L, Regier DA: Utilization of health and mental health services: Three epidemiologic catchment area sites. *Arch Gen Psychiatry* 41:971–978, 1984.

Shepherd M, Cooper B, Brown A: *Psychiatric Illness in General Practice.* London, Oxford University Press, 1966.

Shine D, Demas P: Knowledge of medical students, residents and attending physicians about opiate abuse. *J Med Educ* 59:501–507, 1984.

Smith GR, Monson RA, Ray DC: Psychiatric consultation in somatization disorder: A randomized controlled study. *New Engl J Med* 314:1407–1413, 1986a.

Smith GR Jr., Monson RA, Ray DC: Patients with multiple unexplained symptoms: Their characteristics, functional health, and health care utilization. *Arch Intern Med* 146:6972, 1986b.

Stam M, Strain JJ: Refusal of treatment: The role of psychiatric consultation. *Mt Sinai J Med* 52:4–9, 1985.

Strain JJ: Noncompliance. In: *Psychological Interventions in Medical Practice*. New York, Appleton-Century-Crofts, 1978.

Strain JJ: Letter to the editor re: Clinical and cost benefits of liaison psychiatry. *Amer J Psychiatry* 138:1636–1637, 1981.

Strain JJ, Grossman S: *Psychological Care of the Medically Ill: A Primer in Liaison Psychiatry.* Appleton-Century-Crofts, New York, 1975.

Strain JJ, Hamerman D: Ombudsmen (medical-psychiatric) rounds. An approach to meeting patient-staff needs. *Ann Int Med* 88:550–555, 1978.

Strain JJ, Gise LH, Houpt J, et al.: Mental health training for primary care physicians. Final report, NIMH Contract No. OD-82-0015, 1983.

Strain JJ, Hammer JS, Lyons J, Fahs M, Lebovits A: Cost offset from the psychiatric liaison intervention for elderly hip fracture patients. In: *Abstracts: Physician in the 21st Century; New Paradigms to Cope with Specialization and to Promote Health.* Seventeenth European Conference on Psychosomatic Research, Marburg, West Germany, September 4–9, 1988, p. 207, no. 313.

Thompson TL, II, Stoudemire A, Mitchell WD, et al.: Underrecognition of patients' psychosocial distress in a university hospital medical clinic. *Am J Psychiatry* 140:158, 1983.

Unlenhuth EH, Balter MB, Mellinger GD, et al.: Symptom checklist syndromes in the general population: Correlations with psychotherapeutic drug use. *Arch Gen Psychiatry* 37, 1980.

Utilization Information Services. Albany, NY, Hospital Association of New York State, 1983.

Wallen J: Use of short-term general hospitals by patients with psychiatric diagnoses. Hospital and Cost Utilization Project Research Note 8: DHHS Publication PHS 86-3395. Washington D.C., U.S. Government Printing Office, 1985.

Wallen J, Pincus HA, Goldman HH, et al.: Psychiatric consultations in short-term general hospitals. *Arch Gen Psychiatry* 44:163–168, 1987.

Weschler H, Levine S, Idelson RK, et al.: The physician's role in health promotion: A survey of primary care practitioners. *N Engl J Med* 308:97–100, 1983.

FOUR

Communication

The Key to Becoming Competent and Humane Physicians

LEAH J. DICKSTEIN

> Hippocrates said he "would rather know
> what sort of person has a disease than what
> sort of disease a person has."

The Problem

In the January-February 1988 issue of *The New Physician*, a section entitled "Counts" reads as follows: "Now hear this: 56% of patients believe doctors are not good listeners." An expert on listening, Bob Maidment (1988), commented aptly, "Listening, not talking, is the most used aspect of communication and the least understood. Listening is the underdeveloped other half of talking. We've made the assumption that because most people hear reasonably well, they are also listening. Hearing is a physical process; listening is mental, and they are quite different. The problem is that most of us have very well-developed skills at *faking* listening. We make eye contact, we nod at appropriate times, we agree with the talker and we *hear* most of what is being said, particularly the factual content. But facts alone rarely make up the complete message. The *idea* of what is being expressed, the underlying *theme* of the communication and its context are equally important and may even be more significant than the factual content."

Developing good communication skills is unquestionably basic to the general scientific education and clinical training of competent and humane physicians. Unfortunately, this subject is often delayed or overlooked by medical educators searching for ways to decrease already excessive curricular hours as they simultaneously include in a variety of didactic forms what they perceive as the most current and vital medical knowledge. Furthermore, medical students, eager to learn technical skills enabling them to

54

diagnose diseases and institute effective state-of-the art treatment, assume they possess these acquired communication skills or ignore and are, in fact, unaware of the inadequate quality of their communication. In addition, they do not recognize the distinction and common conflicts between verbal and nonverbal communication. Even more unsettling is the continued unspoken lesson, more by example than by lecture, of a minority of faculty and resident teachers for whom communication with patients and with students is a way to abuse power and authority. Cost containment has also affected medical students' learning to communicate. With most patients' hospitalizations cut short, opportunities to develop deeper relationships have decreased.

Excellent communication skills are often not given much weight in the admissions process. To add to the ever-increasing amount of facts to be learned, and perhaps to predict students' academic success, medical school admissions committees still weigh most heavily applicants' grades in science courses and on MCAT exams. However, several schools in the past few years, including the Johns Hopkins University and the University of Pennsylvania Schools of Medicine, have chosen not to require MCAT scores. Their admissions committees prefer to depend more on students' undergraduate records, personal recommendations, and interviews. Klein and Mumford (1978) offered their "bent twig" hypothesis, which essentially reiterates what has just been stated, i.e., that "the medical school selection process that identifies smart, achievement-oriented, rather aloof persons who know how to get good grades, indirectly gives preference to qualities that frequently accompany a strong premedical background: intense competitiveness, intellectual narrowness and occasional difficulties in getting along with others."

A 1987 survey of 124 deans of U.S. medical colleges (Wickersham 1987) revealed that "because increasing technical skills require less interpersonal skills, today's graduates are no better than their counterparts of fifteen years ago at communicating effectively with their patients," according to 52 percent of the respondents.

Vicki Darrow, class of 1987, University of Washington School of Medicine and OSR (AAMC's Organization of Student Representatives) chair, stated in the spring, 1987 OSR Report (Darrow 1987) that "Programs devoted to communications and ethics have become essential to physicians' education, but many students and faculty remain skeptical about their utility."

Research Evidence

Many educators have long been concerned about physicians' communication skills. Doyle and Ware (1977) identified patient dissatisfaction due in large measure to poor physician conduct, primarily the criterion of caring rather than of competence. Jensen (1981) outlined problems in the doctor-patient relationship with particular emphasis on patients' doubts concerning doctors' interest in them, in their problems, and the seemingly, and perhaps real, impersonal attitude the physicians generally conveyed. Koos found that 64 percent of 1,000 randomly selected families were dissatisfied with their doctor-patient relationship. In 1955 Kasteler et al. found that 48 percent of 328 upper-income and 37 percent of lower-income families changed physicians because they were displeased with the physician's personal qualities (Koos 1955). Finally, Korsch et al. (1968), after questioning 800 mothers about contacts with their children's pediatricians, found that fewer than 7 percent of mothers questioned the physicians' technical competence but 24 percent were dissatisfied with their interpersonal interaction with these physicians.

Although the problem of poor communication and its solution of improved communication seem evident, in actuality this recognition and resolution have not usually occurred. In separate studies, Carkhuff, Berensen, Khajari and Hekmat have shown that empathy decreases as medical technology learning increases (Carkhuff and Berensen 1982). In a *JAMA* special section, "A Piece of My Mind," Sontag (1988), as the attending physician, relates a poignant clinical vignette showing that empathy decreases as medical technology learning increases.

> A symptomatic patient had normal test results but needed empathy and a physician to talk to rather than procedures. Although the trainee health team of resident, intern and student became aware of the patient's needs, only the woman intern responded appropriately at the time. Even several months later, to the attending's dismay, the resident and student were primarily concerned about the technical aspects causing the patient's death rather than about the emotional support the intern had given, which was all that had been needed.

According to reports by the Project on the Status and Education of Women, there are a number of special communication issues pertaining to gender differences (Hall and Sandler 1984). For example, "Teachers may interrupt women more frequently than men or allow them to be interrupted by others in class" or on rounds and in case conferences. "Many faculty are not as likely to call directly on women as on men during class (and clinical) discussion. Professors may often ask questions followed by eye-contact with men students only, as if only men were expected to respond." Unfortunately, instances of subtle and direct gender discrimination are not rare and are committed by those who should know better, i.e., faculty and residents. What should not be overlooked is that this discrimination may be carried out by women faculty and residents as well as by men (Hall 1986).

If miscommunication is allowed to continue between men and women faculty and students, then men students learn from their mentors and role models and may perpetuate the patterns, not only with their peers but with women patients.

Brent and Beckett (1986), in a laudable effort to study medical students' response patterns during patient interviews, used systematic, quantitative observations to measure common response patterns of 68 all-male freshmen in their early twenties. Students' behavior with patients was obtained from audiotaped patient interviews the students had completed during a course in communication and interviewing. Results indicated that students demonstrated a problem common to all patient interviews, i.e., the need for the health professional to provide direction and control over the interview while remaining responsive to the patient.

Four patterns of student interviews emerged:

1. *Questioning facilitators.* These students provided structured questions and facilitative comments to convey their responsiveness to patients.

2. *Prompters.* These students asked more open-ended questions and facilitated concise, rather than narrative, statements.

3. *Declaring facilitators.* These students facilitated narrative patient statements and responded to narrative and concise statements with their own statements. They infrequently used questions which researchers rated as indicating less control over the interview than the other groups.

4. *Elaborators.* These students rarely used facilitation or open-ended questions to indicate their responsiveness to patients, yet they displayed an unusual tendency to respond with statements to patients' concise statements. Interestingly, the researchers stated that they had no basis to assess the relative merits of the different patterns.

The authors do refer to the work of Adler et al. (1970), however, which showed that extensive use of direct questions may reduce the quality of information patients will offer because patients often assume that doctors want only the information they ask about. Adler et al. noted that extensive use of direct questions may also increase both physician authority and patient passivity. As mentioned initially, physicians' deft use of power and authority must be balanced with sensitive regard to patients' healthy use of power in their illness experience.

Brent and Beckett (1986) raise interesting points sometimes overlooked. One is that these student patterns remain stable and are characteristic of particular students. Other researchers state that the interaction patterns of a student may differ, depending on patient variables such as the patient's diagnosis, age or sex; on student variables such as the student's undergraduate major, sex or experience, or simple professional trial, error and wise maturation.

DiMatteo et al. (1979) studied 69 residents and their patients and found that patient satisfaction correlated significantly with the house staff's ability to accurately decode nonverbal communication such as body posture, movement, and facial expressions. In two separate studies, residents' patients were interviewed by others. Patients were found to prefer physicians who could understand their feelings even when they are not able or willing to express such feelings verbally. Burnett and Thompson (1986), writing from the London Hospital Medical College in England, stress that most medical students have very different social and educational backgrounds from those of their patients in the "socially-deprived areas of large cities." Certainly this sociocultural difference may occur for U.S. medical students and must be acknowledged and dealt with constructively in a proactive mode early in the medical education process and again in orientations to clinical rotations.

Furthermore, students are likely to be unconsciously aware but need direct affirmation from their teachers that they will encounter patients whose backgrounds differ from their own. Students must learn to accommodate to their patients' different needs, competencies, and possible lack of specific information or understanding related to the illness and reason for professional contact.

Barlund (1976) also identified students' lack of understanding of lifestyles and levels of the general public's basic medical knowledge. He corroborated other investigators' findings that this is an important factor contributing to poor doctor-patient communication and inevitably leads to misconceptions and misperceptions about patients as individuals.

During preclinical years, in science courses with theoretical constructs, many minute factors must successfully be learned, grasped, and "given back" on successive examinations as proof of competency to become a physician. While it would be ludicrous to state that one doesn't need many facts to practice good medicine, clearly what should also be included in the curriculum is sufficient time and appropriate settings for students to refine their abilities to think, analyze, and grasp both the big and the little picture of their patients' medical situations. Related to this is what Dan (1988) describes in alarm as the repetitive questioning in narrow areas of a student's knowledge and competency base, which he noted on the 1987 MCAT he took out of personal interest, having passed this exam in 1969.

As Dan describes it, this national exam experience presents a first introduction of organized medicine to potential medical students and nowhere in the exam is there any indication of humanitarianism. In fact, in and during the test, students are repeatedly warned against any form of cheating. They in turn continue to talk about "facts they forgot, despite the Kaplan course and that expense," even as they enter the exam room!

A well-known science writer, Morton Hunt, describes his and others' experiences in the patient role and how this role affects one's ability to think and reason logically (Hunt 1988). Hunt offers a vignette:

> A social worker described her obviously incorrect description of an amount of water which was placed in a cup and then poured into a test tube. She stated that even at the time she knew the correct answer yet reacted like a small child with a simplistic, incorrect one.

If students were made aware that this different mental/cognitive experience for their patients stems from the sick role experience itself, they could rationally adjust their communication methods to the reality of patients' changed perceptions and reactions. They could constructively allow for these common discrepancies in perspective and perception, and certainly in increased dependency and regression to a seemingly childish state, typical in many patients.

An additional point to be noted is that until recently women in the patient role and men in the physician role have related to each other as child to adult. Sixty-year-old women were called "Honey" and "Mary" by doctors often young enough to be their sons or grandsons, yet the physicians were called Dr. Smith and Dr. Jones. With consciousness raised as a result of the women's movement, more women patients have assumed an adult stance and participated to a greater extent in their own care and decision-making regarding treatment options. This change has forced men and women physicians to interact differently with women patients. Medical students must also learn that men patients need more encouragement than they have received in the past to reveal fears and symptoms they were raised to "tough out." Many physicians now make concerted efforts to decrease what might be labeled broad inappropriate control over patients. They choose instead to disseminate information and options, and where appropriate, share in decision-making processes.

Medical Students

Before proposing curricular modifications and other options that can enhance medical students' communication skills with patients, not simply for clerkship grades but for their entire professional careers, it is important that discussion focus on medical students themselves as people in context, over time and in familiar as well as unfamiliar environments.

Studies of sex-role socialization along gender lines demonstrate rather clearly that, even before the time of their conception, boys and girls are communicated about and with differently. Parents bring gender-specific sociocultural expectations to their imminent offspring. For example, more than a decade ago researchers determined that, handed the baby in one instance wrapped in a blue blanket and in the next instance in a pink one, men and women subjects told "this is Mary" (in pink) and "this is John" (in blue) gave consistent gender-specific responses. The baby boy was jostled freely with glee and with words to the effect that "he's got strong legs and arms, good for a football player," while comments about the girl baby can be summarized as "what tiny, delicate fingers and toes; she's so pretty" as the subjects held her carefully and protectively! Gifts to the hospital nursery still follow established expectations: dolls for the girls to love, feed, care for, and talk to; trucks, balls, and bats for the boys to control and express their active nonverbal power. Other studies found that girl babies were talked to more and boy babies were allowed to cry longer before being picked up. Preschool boys are still rather consistently told to "keep a stiff upper lip" or "fight back" and suppress, contain, and deny tears and sad, vulnerable feelings so "you won't be called a sissy," while little girls still receive solace, love, hugs, and a cookie as rewards when they succumb with tears to hurt and sad feelings, but they are not usually taught or encouraged to express anger or assertiveness.

These gender-specific, stereotypic communication patterns based on sex role socialization continue as young women and men mature. Women make close friends on a verbal basis and enjoy time to "gossip" and also make time to "just talk" through elementary, junior, and senior high school, college and beyond. Men are encouraged to play on competitive teams to win, boast, and achieve through power moves and the games' rules, but they rarely share personal feelings, particularly of vulnerability, though comparing a continuum of successes is legitimate and expected. In adolescence, women experience conflict over developing and achieving personal goals versus pleasing men so the latter will ask them out on a date and eventually to marry. For the men, raised to accept that actions speak louder than words, unspoken rules are: win high school and college letters for sports, earn academic awards, obtain part-time jobs and first cars, and give flowers and rings to your girls to *show* love rather than to just *talk more*. No wonder, when given the opportunity to hide behind medicine's increasing technology, lab data, and diseased organs, many men easily and unthinkingly fit comfortably into this new yet old mold!

Today's medical students might easily be alluded to as "the microwave generation." They live in an environment in which time is measured in "instants." This revised definition of time must be acknowledged and incorporated into lessons about communication. For example, students not only feed themselves hot dinners cooked in seconds, but they learn about seconds of laser surgery and about epidermal growth factor speeding up healing. When seconds are applied to communication with patients born in different decades, students' awareness must be raised. To understand their patients, they must learn about time in the era of World War I, the 1920s, the 1930s, World War II, the 1940s, and the 1950s. Along with instant technology, students need to learn about human patience!

Recent Demographic Changes

One should raise several points against generalizing that most students fit a narrow, stereotypic description, particularly since 1982, when the number of twenty-two-year-old white male applicants to medical schools first began to decrease. Since then, increasing numbers of women and more mature, second-career men and women students have filled the vacant places. These students have brought different personality characteristics to the medical environment. Women, with more verbal facility from the time they learn to speak and sex-role socialized to please and relate to others as a prime life focus regardless of the type of work they choose, have been noted to be more empathetic and to spend more time with all patients (Shapiro 1987). Because it is really "second-nature" for them to speak empathetically to others, they seem to do it spontaneously and well. For different reasons, the second-career men who choose to return to the medical student role bring with them work and life experiences which, although at work may have brought financial success, left these men feeling unfulfilled. Many of them state just that: "I want to help people and work with them directly. I want to make a difference in people's lives and not simply by selling x-ray equipment or serving as legal counsel to businesses." Now in their late twenties, thirties, and early forties, these men were socialized earlier and perhaps pressured to compete and gain personal power and success. In medical school they allow their "feminine" traits to surface since these were thwarted in their childhoods and youth when the men were taught to "keep a stiff upper lip." Generally, these men relate extremely well to their patients.

Furthermore, although a certain percentage of the most academically gifted, typical medical students have not participated in undergraduate extracurricular activities, the majority have. They have made time to do hospital volunteer work to demonstrate and confirm interest in their future careers to admissions committees and to themselves, but they have also participated in other extracurricular activities for personal satisfaction and maturation and because they enjoy the company of others.

Meeting their cadavers on "day one" of school, along with receiving overwhelming numbers of handouts to integrate with voluminous lecture and student-transcribed notes, too many students may be immediately "redirected" away from their sincere interest in "talking to" patients. Most find it quite advantageous to focus solely on amassing factual details. Whether they attend class or not, the majority of students pay for transcribed notes because lecturers' rates of talking often overtake their ability to write. Unfortunately, by their sophomore year, a sizable proportion of students, including even those most academically proficient, intermittently refrain from attending class because they find their independent library study hours more profitable for test scores than sitting and listening to lecturers. These experiences account in part for the "dehumanizing effect" attributed to the usual preclinical educational experience.

Faculty, even those with moderate clinical teaching experience, attest to the fact that frequently medical students with the least scientific knowledge among the members of the ward medical team obtain the most complete pertinent histories because these students spend time with, listen effectively, observe carefully, clarify clearly, and talk to their patients. Patients are aware that these young student doctors don't know everything, yet they appreciate the time, attention, and, most importantly, the "listening ear and observant eye" of "their" student doctor, and so share more than with "those in long white coats," residents and attendings, who too often appear restless, preoccupied, curt, and exhausted and simply fly in, by, and out, not giving patients time to ask or tell them anything that would take more than fifteen seconds.

Another aspect of communication needs mention. Usually medical students refer to their patients as "Mr. Smith" and "Mrs. Jones"; that is, until attempting to imitate a minority of their resident role models, some begin referring to "the cancer in Room 105" or to "the one in bed three in Room 214" or to different, disenfranchised patient populations, in stereotypic, derogatory terms.

Necessity for Good Communication

Korsch et al. (1968) found that patients who verbalized satisfaction with their medical treatment also felt doctors communicated satisfactorily and understood patients' concerns.

In 1973, Fletcher emphasized the ideal paradigm "that for optimal benefit, effective communication must depend on an understanding by doctors of the patient as an individual who has an illness, rather than as a disease process alone." He stressed that both information-gathering from, and its delivery to, the patient must be matched to the patient's knowledge, social background, interest, and needs.

If faculty shared with students the important fact that the primary cause for a large percentage of malpractice suits relates to poor and/or lack of empathetic communication from physicians to patients, realistically, students might be more motivated to retain the personal humanism they brought to medical school (Blum 1960). In recent years, countless analyses have been made of the reasons for the proliferation of lawsuits against physicians in practice, and the "communication factor" is always included. Experienced clinicians, sensitive to patients' reactions, readily admit that their constructive communication greatly affects patient compliance (Hulka et al. 1966).

After thirty-five hours on call, a resident described her anxiety dreams centering around feeling unprepared to deal with the constantly new emergencies she faced (Chavez 1988). The importance of this resident's admitting to concern about her competency is that during awake on-call hours, residents' attitudes toward students and time to interact with and teach them clearly depends a great deal on their own self-image and self-worth. If residents in turn could allow themselves to share the newness of their own physician roles, including the concomitant understandable anxiety and apprehension they must acknowledge in order to deal with ongoing life and death challenges they face, then resident-student communication would improve, be more of a teaching-learning experience for the dyad, and finally result in better care for patients and team-building for residents and students.

As child abuse, drug, and alcohol problems, along with suicide and suicidal potential and sexually transmitted diseases, escalate across the spectrum of patients, medical students must communicate effectively to gain information when patients seek treatment. Gaining pertinent information in such cases certainly takes more skill than getting responses about measles or rheumatic fever. Relating supportively and effectively to parents of newborns also demands extraordinary sensitivity.

Those choosing psychiatry must similarly be skilled communicators in order to deal with other mental health colleagues, all health professionals, and the myriad of signs and symptoms defining disorders that were unrecognized less than a decade ago.

Increased technology doesn't negate the need for effective communication; in fact, it actually increases it. With more elective medical options, not only elective surgery but elective fertility and other medical treatments including life and death decisions and care for the terminally ill, competent interpersonal physician-patient communication becomes the core of medical practice. With increased openness across most of society, communication to the physician may entail topics, confessions, and requests for treatment that never have been verbalized outside the bedroom and confessional.

Burn-out occurs among many physicians in many specialties. Whether in oncology, infectious disease such as AIDS, or geriatrics, those who work with the terminally ill must recognize their human potential and responsibility to be the bulwark for the dying and for their significant others, offering empathy yet reserving enough to sustain themselves over their career decades.

Students must become aware that people in their care, their patients, are dependent upon the students because of their professional role and that dependency creates a vulnerability to losing human dignity and integrity simply because of illness. Therefore, it really is a necessity, and not a choice, that physicians become aware of their own values and attitudes, and simultaneously that they understand patients' attitudes, values, and personal life goals.

Suggested Solutions

Weihs and Chapados (1986) found that a structured ten-week course on the development of specific interviewing skills for first-year medical students proved to be beneficial. The patient-centered medical interview is effective with careful analysis of signs and symptoms, an understanding of patients' feelings about their condition, and the implications of their illness for daily life (Weihs and Chapados, 1986).

The Developmental Helping Model of Carkhuff (1983), based on the client-centered theories of Carl Rogers, teaches skills which include attending and responding. Patients perceive students as possessing the core conditions of empathy, nonpossessive warmth, and genuineness.

In discussing the contributions of ethics and psychology to medicine, Bergsma and Thomasma (1985) outline what they describe as "first level," important relevant factors, that is, the most concrete, consisting of measured numbers of verbal and nonverbal interactions.

They designate "second level" as that of therapeutic success. They describe their research which showed that "the greater the degree of information and possibly personal engagement between professionals, patients and their families prior to surgical operations, the fewer the subsequent side effects experienced by the patients" (Skipper and Leonard 1985). They define "third level" as that of attitudes and values which center around the way people compare their own illness with others' to make themselves more exceptional and unique.

An excellent program has existed at Utrecht University School of Medicine in the Netherlands since 1984, based on work by Gerritsma and Betenburg (see Betenburg and Gerritsma, 1983). Interactional analyses of student-patient relationships are used, in which patient-actors are trained to give feedback to students. Lila M. Wallis developed the Teaching Associates Program at Cornell University Medical College in response to women medical students' requests to learn correctly how to perform breast and pelvic exams. Men students folowed with requests to learn how to perform male genitorectal exams correctly. Dr. Wallis hired and trained women and men "associates" to serve simultaneously as subjects in the patient role and as instructors to teach medical students correct techniques by communicating clear feedback of their correct and incorrect verbal and nonverbal techniques in history-taking and physical examination. This nationally recognized and successful program has served as a model to more than 85 U.S. and Canadian medical schools since 1979 (Wallis 1988). For the last several years, an annual national Teaching Associates meeting is held so that Dr. Wallis can share her program with faculty and students.

In 1987, an issue of *The New Physician* contained an article by a medical student describing her interaction with a supposedly comatose patient. All health staff who came in contact with the patient had simply performed their tasks. But this medical student as she performed her duties spoke to the patient about having to draw her blood, obtain blood gases, about the weather, family, and her feelings. When the patient regained consciousness, she verbalized her gratitude to the student for this communication and caring, which was unique and very meaningful despite the patient's inability at the time to respond.

With their similar programs, Gerritsma and Betenburg in Utrecht and Wallis in New York proved that it is possible to clarify behavior for medical students (and physicians) in such a way that they become aware of the kind of behavior they use, and the effects this behavior has on their interactions with patients.

Tazelaar (1980), on the other hand, demonstrated the difficulty of really influencing and changing attitudes. Others described the "autonomous physician" who "learned" communication skills, and who behaves like an actor in an ill-fitting role, which is noticed by everyone. Unquestionably behavior alone is not enough to communicate effectively; appropriate attitude must accompany it.

In *The New Physician*, March 1988, Timothy Flynn recounts an experience about miscommunication under difficult circumstances for a medical resident during an on-call night. He was called to see what he assumed was a "typically demanding and difficult geriatric patient," who, he further assumed, had minor problems, only to discover she was his 80-year-old, independent, generous, vivacious and caring former landlady. Her hospital behavior, which he had generalized to be her usual personality before he recognized who the patient was, stemmed from her "mask of illness." Scarcely can there be one among us who has not had the same humbling experience but often not with such a happy outcome!

At Emory University, Cohen-Cole (1985) has developed and written about student training programs in communication skills. Rosen et al. (1985) outline the medical student's major and important role of empathetic listener, supporter, and thorough information-giver in relation to a patient throughout the surgical experience. They describe how this interaction can definitely affect surgical outcome.

Another excellent example of teaching effective physician-patient communication to medical students occurs through the "Medical Students As Partners" program at the University of Missouri–Kansas City School of Medicine. Developed by Duckwall et al. (1987), the program matches junior students with seniors, and the team leader is a physician-scholar "docent," who teaches and supervises the student team of 12 and serves as attending physician for the team's patients. The unique feature of this teaching model, apart from the obvious teamwork, friendship, support systems, and eased transition to the clinician role, is that it offers students ongoing lessons in physician-patient communication from role models they get to know well.

The Profile of Nonverbal Sensitivity (the PONS) test of Rosenthal and Hall is a useful preclinical technique in teaching interviewing. The PONS is a reliable 45-minute, 16-mm film test of an individual's ability to decode accurately another's body movements, facial expression, and voice-tone cues of emotion.

For the more mature student who is a parent, communication earlier in the patient's treatment process can be easier. Student-parents, if they have not themselves been ill, may have cared for their sick children and learned to tolerate regressive behavior, realizing it is temporary and related to helplessness, fear, pain, and the unknown. Most likely, more mature students have also dealt with ill parents or elderly relatives, and these experiences can facilitate their communication with patients. It is almost axiomatic for preclinical faculty to reassure entering older students to do the best they can and to predict that freshman grades will improve as they settle in to the full-time student role as sophomores. Predictably, older students' life experiences often enable them to "shine" when they enter clinical rotations and seem able to assume a variety of new simultaneous responsibilities with relative ease, including relating to all health team members.

Another aspect of communication which must be elucidated is that there are new frontier areas for physicians and patients to confer about which did not exist a decade or two ago. These subjects relate to biomedical ethics, life-support system decisions, organ donation, treatment choices, and the many new technologies, in vitro fertilization among others (Veatch 1980).

Some students are likely to find themselves involved in notifying families of patients' deaths or to respond to directions to meet families in a hospital waiting room to request their permission to perform an autopsy. Medical technologies have advanced so quickly and so far that life and death matters students may be asked to communicate about to both patients and their families are not in textbooks. These crises often are also not seen as important enough to discuss as separate proactive issues by attendings and residents, who feel pressured themselves to deal simply with the urgent decision which resulted from the student's communication with the family. Residents and attendings focus instead on family-involved issues of whether to pull life supports, to allow kidneys to be retrieved or to perform an enucleation for an eye bank. Students, imitating their role models, often are unaware of the momentous decisions they are involved in and asked to get answers to, from uninformed, or at least not well-informed, and certainly traumatized patients' families.

In the regular *JAMA* column "A Piece of My Mind," one entitled "Self-Defense" concerns a third-year female medical student's dilemma, universal to all current clinical students, of remaining empathic to a dying AIDS patient, a man who "no longer appears human because of the blood oozing from lesions all over his body." She describes how her response changed from an initial hovering with ice, Ensure, and cookies she'd baked, to beginning to be unresponsive to his incessant cry of "Hello; is anyone there?" His plea for understanding and compassion drew her increasing unresponsiveness because she felt she had no hope to offer him and without outside guidance thought her only choice was to withdraw. (Friedman 1987)

As medical educator-clinicians, we must develop ways to cope with our own helplessness, hopelessness, and ultimate acceptance in response to our dying patients. Then we must teach students to do the same in responsible fashion without becoming inured, suffering professional burn-out or seeming preoccupied as defenses against these situations (Lehman 1983).

One medical student described her fear, trepidation, and loneliness going into and surviving her own surgery, without being spoken to or told anything by anyone until the night following the morning surgery. Then a medical student, on call for the night, after checking her vital signs and wound, gently held her hand and softly said, "Everything's fine." He then waited for her to speak and ask about her condition.

Another area of patient-physician communication which is often overlooked is that of helplessness with the violent, acutely out-of-control, homicidal or suicidal patient. A protocol of questions and comments, which alternately may provoke a patient to lose control, or communication which might return a patient's control, should be presented and discussed during the clerkship orientation as well as in more specific proactive discussions of Alzheimer's disease, crack use, diabetic insulin instability, the DTs of alcohol abuse and paranoid psychosis, to cite just a few common crisis situations (Barash 1984).

Effective communication is also needed in the areas of complex cardiac surgeries. Students involved in history-taking preoperatively who follow patients through surgery and the postoperative transitional stages to discharge must be taught how and what specific fears and feelings to broach with patients who may simply appear generally anxious, depressed, sleepless, or even psychotic, and unaware of their reactive feelings (Layne and Yudofsky 1971).

Another 1980s addendum to the list of situations calling for clear and humane communication from medical students to patients is that concerning informed consent with its therapeutic and legal issues. Medical school applicants' general wish to "treat patients" differs greatly from the multilayered approach students must learn to use with patients, particularly in the increasing number of clinical situations in which there is choice of treatments, with one not superior to another, and where final outcomes may be equally uncertain. Students must be guided beyond a goal of solely comprehending the pathophysiology of drug treatment. They must be informed clearly and continually that there are humane issues involved for patients in each and every encounter with treatment protocols. Young professionals must be taught not to ignore this equally important aspect of treatment.

An often overlooked issue in communication involves students identifying who they are to patients, families, and significant others. Are they simply physicians, or must they state directly their student status? Although guidelines from the federal government and Joint Commission on the Accreditation of Hospitals say that patients should be informed about the status of caregivers, this ruling is not always followed. One study revealed that only 37.5 percent of teaching hospitals inform patients routinely that medical students will be involved in their care, 83 percent of medical schools provide students with instruction about patient interaction, and only 51 percent insisted that students introduce themselves as such (Wessen, 1966).

Just as all medical students complete a preclinical course in the behavioural sciences and a clinical psychiatry rotation, they need further reinforcement regarding how their own personalities and life experiences impact on their physician roles with patients. The concepts of intrapsychic transference and countertransference must be explained far in advance of psychiatry lectures in practical and obvious terms, as foreseen experiences for all physicians regardless of level of training or specialty. In addition, students need guidance and assistance to deal with their transference and countertransference feelings beyond their understanding of interpersonal theories of personality and behavior, family systems, affect and cognition so that appropriate empathy and consequent communication are maintained.

Discussion and Conclusion

In addition to requirements for computer literacy among medical students for their academic success and future professional lives, and beyond requirements for physicians to make diagnoses by television-telephone hookup, medical students must be taught how to communicate directly, verbally and nonverbally with patients, and they must be evaluated on their competencies to do so. Effective communication skills must include effective listening, analysis of what is said and not said, observation of body language, and clarification by the interviewer with the patient of what the patient has said.

Ideally this teaching must begin on the first day of medical school and continue to the last day. The teaching must take many forms, but unquestionably should include demonstration by faculty. From the inception, faculty must interview patients with students present, in small groups and large, on every service and in every clinical setting and situation. Overextended faculty must accept this primary responsibility to demonstrate by example all the subtleties of effective, humane communication with patients and their significant others in emergency rooms, clinics, ICUs, and all situations where taking a history, showing respect, tact, trust, honesty, understanding, thoroughness, medical knowledge, and patience make the difference between someone's life and death.

Time must be made each year of medical school and on every rotation for attendings to discuss the practical and painful aspects of patients' dying, because an elective during preclinical years on the issues of death and dying is not the same, but in fact is only an introduction to the life of a physician.

With newly recognized illnesses such as panic disorder, social phobia, and AIDS, physicians cannot always turn to their teachers for years of experience because their experience may not be much greater. In relating to geriatric patients, including the "oldest old," those over 80 and the frail elderly, some afflicted with Alzheimer's disease, communication skills must be specific and supported with enormous patience and humanity, not only for this group of patients but also for their exhausted families.

Needless to say, medical students need teachers who model effective communication, not only with patients but with students themselves. Inquiring of students as individuals how they are, how they feel, how their lives are currently, and their plans for the future serve more than apparent uses. Students learn that physicians can be humane professionals as well as skilled and knowledgeable narrowly focused technocrats. Faculty outreach to students can lessen student stress and therefore increase learning; it can also serve as excellent role-modeling for students to relate to their patients.

Ordinary people are expected to do extraordinary things. Yet when goals are refined, the overriding objective is to teach students that they must combine the power of the physician with the needs of the patient, and there must be straightforward, humane understanding between the two.

The media and many articles in medical journals increasingly question the quality of current medical care, and the growing perception of the public is that quality is a problem. Through Medicare hospital mortality statistics and organized medicine's tort reform campaigns, physicians are to be judged on how good their clinical results are and how cost-efficient their practices are, enabling patients to select physicians by these criteria. However, unless physician-patient communication is directly addressed during medical school, quality can never be equated synonymously with care.

Some physicians contend that the third-party insurance system has effectively ended the empathic physician-patient relationship of the past through its erosion of physician authority by government regulators' and third-party payers' control of practice style, including availability of personal physicians, on-call schedules, and freedom for physicians to practice medicine with the best interest of patients foremost in mind.

Another important, though overlooked, consideration related to physician-patient communication is that physicians must teach patients how to communicate with them. Clearly, if medical students learn how to teach patients to communicate well and completely, students will learn more and be able to help patients more. Students must be taught how to teach their patients how to ask questions, how to describe symptoms, how to feel comfortable sharing feelings and experiences never before told to anyone, how to ask for help, solace and advice, not just for pain pills. Students must be taught that for them and for their patients all questions are appropriate, and that asking questions improves students' learning and patients' treatment. Finally, in this regard students and their patients must learn that the last question every physician must ask is, "Is there anything I haven't asked about that you think I should know?" Then the student-physician should remain silent to allow the patient time to gather courage to respond, perhaps about bloody stool, breast lump, history of incest or alcohol abuse, or even, "Am I going to die soon?"

Increasing numbers of useful methods of teaching students how to communicate professionally have evolved at different schools developed by caring and creative faculty. One method that might prove useful and satisfying, in addition to the use of videotapes, role models, and simulated patients, would be to assign every entering freshman a child and its family from the well-baby clinic and an elderly resident from a nursing home or senior citizen apartment complex. S. Spafford Ackerly, first chair of psychiatry at the University of Louisville in the 1930s, attempted to initiate a program such as this during the early years of his tenure with medical students and children.

Students should be introduced to their patients *before* they meet their cadavers the first week of school. Students should keep diaries of weekly contacts during their four years of medical school and discuss their experiences at once-monthly meetings with their "physician-supervisors" also assigned for four years. These supervisors could be responsible for several freshmen and guide the development of humane communication skills in young physicians through group supervision without regard for primary medical responsibilities, which would *not* be assumed.

Effective and complete communication is a major key to serving as competent, humane physicians. As teachers, we are responsible to ensure that students possess this key.

REFERENCES

Adler, L. M., Ware, J. E., Enelow, A. J.: "Changes in Medical Interviewing Style after Instruction with Two Closed-Circuit Television Techniques." *Journal of Medical Education* 1970; 4:221.

Barlund, D. C.: "The Mystification of Meaning: Doctor-Patient Encounters." *Journal of Medical Education* 1976; 1:716–725.

Barash, D.: "Diffusing the Violent Patient before He Explodes." *RN Journal*, March 1984, pp. 11–15.

Batenburg, V., Gerritsma, G. J. M.: "Interviewing: Initial Student Problems." *Journal of Medical Education* 1983; 17:235–239.

Bergsma, J., Thomasma, D. C.: "The Contribution of Ethics and Psychology to Medicine." *Social Science and Medicine* 1985; 20(7):745–752.

Blum, R. H.: *The Management of the Doctor-Patient Relationship.* McGraw-Hill, New York, 1960.

Brent, E. E., Beckett, D. E.: "Common Response Patterns of Medical Students in Interviews of Hospitalized Patients." *Medical Care* 1986; 24(11):981–989.

Burnett, A. C., Thompson D. G.: "Aiding the Development of Communication Skills in Medical Students." *Medical Education* 1986; 20:424–431.

Carkhuff, R. R.: *Interpersonal Skills and Human Productivity.* Human Resources Development Press, Amherst, Mass., 1983.

Carkhuff, R., Berensen, B.: *Beyond Counseling and Therapy.* Holt, Rinehart and Winston, New York, 1967.

Chavez, A.: "Night after Call, My Perspective." *New Physician* 1988; 37(3):17.

Cohen-Cole, S: In *New Physician*, November 1985.

Dan, B.: "MCAT: Desperately Seeking Med School." *JAMA* 1988; 259(3):405–407.

Darrow, V.: *OSR Report*, Spring 1987.

Dickstein, L. J.: "Social Change and Dependency in University Men: The White Knight Complex Unresolved." *Journal of College Student Psychotherapy* 1986; 1:31–41.

DiMatteo, M. R., Freidman, H. S., Taranta, A: "Sensitivity to Bodily Communication as a Factor in Practitioner-Patient Rapport." *Journal of Nonverbal Behavior* 1979; 1:18–26.

Doyle, B. J., Ware, J. E.: "Physician Conduct and Other Factors That Affect Consumer Satisfaction with Medical Care." *Journal of Medical Education* 1977; 52:793–801.

Duckwall, J., Arnold, L., Willoughby, T. C., Calkins, V., Hamburger, S.: "Innovations in Medical Education." Exhibits, AAMC Group on Medical Education, 1987.

Enelow, A. J., Swisher, S. N.: *Interviewing and Patient Care.* Oxford University Press, London, 1972.

Friedman, S. J.: "Self-Defense." *JAMA* 1987; 258:34.

Hall, R. M.: "The Campus Climate Revisited: Chilly for Women Faculty, Administrators, and Graduate Students." Project on the Status and Education of Women, Association of American Colleges, Washington, D.C., 1986.

Hall, R. M., Sandler, B. R.,: "The Classroom Climate: A Chilly One for Women." Project on the Status and Education of Women, Association of American Colleges, Washington, D.C., 1982.

Hulka, B., Cassel, J., Kupper, L., Burdetter, J.: "Communication, Compliance, and Concordance between Physicians and Patients with Prescribed Medications." *American Journal of Public Health* 1966; 66:847–853.

Hunt, M.: "Sick Thinking." *New York Times Magazine,* January 1988, pp. 22–23.

Jensen, P. S.: "The Doctor-Patient Relationship: Headed for Impasse or Improvement." *Annals of Internal Medicine* 1981; 95:769–771.

Klein H., Mumford E.: "The Bent Twig: Psychiatry and Medical Education." *American Journal of Psychiatry* 1978; 135:320–324.

Koos, E. L.: "Metropolis: What City People Think of Their Medical Services." *American Journal of Public Health* 1955; 45:1551–1557.

Korsch, B. M., Gozzi, E. K., Francis, V: "Gaps in Doctor-Patient Communication." *Pediatrics* 1968; 42:855–871.

Layne, O. L., Jr., Yudofsky, S. C.: "Post-Operative Psychosis in Cardiology Patients." *New England Journal of Medicine* 1971; 284:518–520.

Lehmann, S.: "Training Personnel in the Prevention and Management of Violent Behavior." *Hospital and Community Psychiatry* 1983; 34:40–43.

Maidment, B.: "Robin's Reader." *For Physicians and Their Patients,* Spring 1988, p. 4.

Nichols, D: "On Call for the Night." *New Physician* 1987; 36(9):21–22.

Rosenthal, R., Hall, J. A., DiMatteo, M. R., Rogers, P. C., Archer, D.: "Sensitivity to Non-Verbal Communications." *The PONS Test,* Johns Hopkins University Press, Baltimore, 1979.

Shapiro, M: *Getting Doctored: Critical Reflections on Becoming a Physician.* New Society Educational Foundation, Santa Cruz, Calif., 1987.

Skipper, J. K., Leonard, R. C.: *Social Interaction and Patient Care.* Lippincott, Philadelphia, 1965.

Sontag, S. J.: "A Piece of My Mind. *JAMA* 1988; 259(7):1070–1071.

Tazelaar, F. "Mental inconquenties-Sociale Restricties," *Diss. Utrecht,* 1980.

Veatch, R. M.: "Professional Ethics: New Principles for Physicians." *Hastings Center Reports* 1980; 10(3):16–19.

Wallis, L: "Teaching Associates Program." *New Physician* 1988; 40(10):20–21.

Weihs, K., Chapados, J. T.: "Interviewing Skills Training—A Study." *Social Science and Medicine* 1986; 23(1):31–34.

Wessen, A.: "Hospital Ideology and Communication between Ward Personnel," in Scott, W. R., Volkart, E. H., *Medical Care.* John Wiley, New York, 1966.

Wickersham, C.: "The Future of Medicine, as Educators See It." *Private Practice,* 1987, pp. 12–23.

The Ideal Physician

Requisite Attitudes, Knowledge, and Skills

HUGH C. HENDRIE

Under the influence of Benjamin Bloom (1976) and others, when modern educators consider teaching objectives they describe knowledge and skill acquisition as well as attitude changes which are measurable and which when present would confirm that the student has realized the course goals. In this chapter, I would like first of all to consider the attitudes, knowledge, and skills in addition to those already assumed in biomedical training which would be desirable for physicians to achieve in order to provide competent and humane comprehensive clinical care. This goal would appear to be mutually acceptable to the medical profession and to society at large and certainly was a pivotal one for Dr. Roeske in her career.

Attitudes

The role of physicians and their value systems has been the subject of widespread public comment over the past several decades. The concern expressed by both professional and lay critics often focuses on the weakening of the traditional doctor-patient relationship and a perceived diminution in humanistic values in physicians in their dealings with patients.

Max Lerner, writing in the *Saturday Review* in 1975, rather succinctly summarized these concerns:

> A case in point is the medical profession which has become a cluster of highly trained specialties in which not only the patient gets lost but also the doctor. A general practitioner used to know less about some things than does the specialist of today but he saw and treated and knew his patient as a whole person and the patient saw him in turn as a whole person. There was little talk of malpractice, little trouble about insurance for doctors and little litigiousness by patients. All of these have come out of the impersonality of the medical relationship today, which in turn has proved a bonanza for lawyers.

These unfortunate developments in medical care have generally been attributed to increasing medical specialization, growth of the modern medical industrial complex, and alteration in the economic basis of medicine with the emergence of the physician as businessperson. As the subtitle for a 1987 *Newsweek* report on medicine stated, "money, machines and politics are changing American doctors and the way they treat you."

There is a tendency in many but by no means all critics (not, for example, Starr 1982) to assume that before the advent of modern technology and business practices there was a golden age of medical practice when physicians consistently adhered to excellent standards of humane care and were held in uniformly high regard by society. However, even the most cursory examination of English literture would make one believe that skepticism about doctors' motivations is not new. A cartoon by the eighteenth-century English caricaturist Robert Dighton (1970), which I sometimes use when discussing medical ethics with medical students, has the legend "How merrily we Doctor's Be / We Humbug the Public and Pocket the Fee." In English fiction there is a long gallery of physician rogues, from the duplicitous if nonpracticing Dr. Blifil in Fielding's *Tom Jones* to the members of the medical profession indicted by A. J. Cronin in *The Citadel,* which brought down the ire of the medical establishment upon its physician-author.

Lest the impression is left from these accounts that physician misbehavior was solely a preoccupation of English-speaking authors, one has only to read Moliere's *Le malade imaginaire.* The servant Toinet, for example, in replying to the lament of Diafoirus that great people expect to be cured by physicians states:

> That's a good jest indeed, and they are very impertinent to expect that you gentlemen should cure 'em; you don't attend them for that purpose; you only go to take your fees and prescribe remedies, tis their business to cure themselves if they can.

Indeed, the use by Moliere and other authors and dramatists of health-related topics as metaphors for societal ills reminds us that it is not always easy to separate doctors' values from prevailing societal mores. Physicians' behavior is shaped by and in turn reflects the culture of which the physicians are a part.

It appears to be true, nonetheless, that public concern about doctors' behavior has intensified as well as changed in focus. There is less societal concern about the physician's ability to cure illness—which, if anything, may be overestimated—as there is an altered expectation of professional behavior, including the behavior of physicians. Patients and their families are now less likely to tolerate the authoritarian attitude of the physician and are requiring a greater degree of openness in their communications with their doctors and a sense of decision sharing in proposed medical care. This sharing (or loss?) of total physician responsibility for medical decisions is seen not only in individual patient-physician interactions but also in greater intervention in medical care by agencies of government and private industry, actions which are often dollar driven.

The medical profession has certainly not been blind to these criticisms. Humanism in medicine has been addressed in many articles in professional journals and discussed in recent symposia, conferences, and commissioned works sponsored by, among others, the Kaiser Family Foundation (White 1988), the Association of American Medical Colleges (Schofield 1984), and the American Board of Internal Medicine (1983).

Part of these deliberations has been a reconsideration of the role of the physician in modern society, the dimensions of which have been obscured somewhat, at least in the eyes of some observers, by the aforementioned overestimation of the efficacy of high technology treatments for individual patients. "As a consequence . . . the recognition of medicine as a system of patient care whose functions are the relief and control of illness is obscured, and the importance of the doctor-patient relations ignored" (Stoekle 1987). The tasks of physicians who provide patient care include diagnosis and treatment of illness, communicating information to the patient about the illness, personal support of the patient throughout the stages of illness including death, maintenance of the chronically ill, and prevention of disease and disability by education and preventive treatment. Clearly, for these expanded functions the attitudes and qualities which should be possessed by physicians assume paramount importance. These qualities have been simply stated by the American Board of Internal Medicine (1983) as integrity, respect, and compassion. Morris Green, in another chapter in this volume, incorporates these values and others in his description of a master clinician.

Perhaps the most elegant restatement of the attitudes of the ideal physician was incorporated in the work of another contributor to this volume, Roger Bulger, when he attempted to update the Hippocratic oath. His first three articles are:

> I promise my patients competence, integrity, candor, personal commitment to their best interests, compassion and absolute discretion and confidentiality within the law. . . . I shall do by my patients as I would be done by. I shall obtain consultation whenever I or they˙desire, shall include them to the extent they wish in all important decisions and shall minimize suffering whenever a cure cannot be obtained, understanding that a dignified death is an important goal in everyone's life. . . . I shall try to establish a friendly relationship with my patients and shall accept each one in a non-judgmental manner appreciating the validity and worth of different value systems and according to each person a full measure of human dignity.

It is difficult to find fault with these ideals even though it is not always easy to perceive methods to inculcate them into our future physicians, given the imperfections of modern society. Obviously the development and maintenance of these values is a lifelong task, starting long before entry into medical school and continuing for the remainder of the physicians' careers. As discussed in other chapters, student experiences in medical school should at least not be counterproductive to the development of these ideals. While introducing courses in humanities and ethics has been proposed as a solution, it is likely that nothing would be so effective as example. Medical students need to be exposed to physicians who in their clinical work possess the qualities described (and exemplified) by Dr. Green, preferably clinicians who may be observed caring for patients over long periods of time. That this is not happening at present in medical schools and the reasons why it is not happening are discussed in other parts of this book.

Knowledge

While the impetus for a reevaluation of doctors' attitudes and value systems has arisen largely from negative factors—i.e., increasing dissatisfaction both inside and outside the medical profession with the practice of high-tech, highly specialized medicine—the stimulus for content change in medical schools derives from the rapid accumulation of knowledge about the parameters of health and disease from the social sciences and neurobiology over the past fifty years.

This information, which is discussed in detail elsewhere in this book, includes (1) the now vast amount of evidence which links environmental factors with health and illness—the relationship between illness prevalence, life expectancy, and infant mortality with broadly determined indicators of social and economic well being; the deleterious effects on health of unemployment, continuous occupational stress, bereavement and early maternal separation; the mediating influence on stress and illness of social support and the availability of close loving relationships; (2) the identification of behavioral risk factors for illness, including smoking, diet, exercise, and sexual behavior; (3) the recently acquired evidence that psychosocial intervention favorably affects disease outcome and can be cost-effective; and (4) the recognition that a large proportion of the work of primary care physicians involves patients with somatically expressed symptoms of distress.

The methods and techniques of the disciplines of epidemiology, medical sociology, psychology, medical anthropology, and biostatistics have undergone a transformation in this century in many ways as remarkable as those of the biological sciences. Rather than being confined to the study of general health and a few specific communicable diseases, they have now been applied with considerable success to the understanding of such complicated and chronic disorders as hypertension and heart disease, cancer, and the major psychiatric disorders, including depression, schizophrenia, and alcoholism. In association with advances in medical genetics, it is likely that this new information will lead to profound alteration in the conceptual models of illness and health as well as to methods of treatment and prevention. Yet, presentations from the behavioral and social sciences do not presently occupy a significant proportion of the medical school curriculum and certainly do not compare in value among most medical students and faculty with contributions from the more traditional basic sciences. This situation, as analyzed by participants at the Wickenburg Conference (White 1988), may be traced to previous decisions that relegated the population-based sciences for the most part to schools of public health, which were separated geographically as well as intellectually from the medical schools in the United states. This isolation was in great contrast to the incorporation of the basic biological sciences into medical school curricula which occurred in the post-Flexner age. As a result, the social sciences and public health "were virtually barred from central roles in the evolution of modern medicine, its theories, practices and educational priorities" (White 1988).

Not that social issues were completely ignored in medical school curricula. For example, in 1912 a course on medical sociology lasting thirty-three hours was taught to junior and senior medical students at the Indiana University School of Medicine. The course outline was as follows:

> A course emphasizing the relation of the patient's home life, of his work, and of his environment to the production of disease and to its treatment. Special attention is given to occupational diseases, to those resulting from poor hygienic conditions in the home or at work and to the influence of worry, poor diet, irregular hours, alcohol, etc. (Indiana University 1912)

The fate of this course is perhaps instructive. It was first listed as under the direction of the chairman of the Department of Internal Medicine. After several years it was the responsibility of the chief of social work and was shortened in length. Finally, around 1929–30, it appears to have been abandoned. Several years later a course entitled Public Health and Preventive Medicine was established which may have assumed some of the topics covered in the medical sociology presentation. In Indiana, as in other U.S. medical schools, courses in behavioral sciences first appeared in the early 1960s.

In addition to formal courses in public health, community health, epidemiology, and preventive medicine, which are taught by some schools, all U.S. medical schools still include in their curriculum courses in the social and behavioral sciences, primarily in the freshman and sophomore years, as well as psychiatric clerkships, which occur in the junior years. A recent survey of medical school curricula by educational assistant Donna Clair revealed that behavioral sciences and related topics occupied an average of ninety-two hours' time in U.S. medical schools in 1987–88. These courses had a variety of labels, including Behavioral Sciences, Ethics, Medical Practice in Society, Social Medicine, Sexuality, Health and Society, Medical Humanities, Family Dynamics, and many others. Although there was considerable variation in the length of these courses and in the position they occupied in the curriculum, most appeared to be isolated and relatively brief, occurring in years otherwise dominated by the intensive study of basic sciences. The utility of these courses, which are usually not well incorporated into the overall medical curriculum, is doubtful. At least one observer of the medical school scene has no doubt: "The behavioral scientists expend a lot of effort trying to attract the attention of the students during their first or second years; however, the results have been disappointing with poor class attendance in many schools" (Scholfield 1984). What is clear from the wide variety even in titles of these courses is that there is no consensus in medical schools as to what this material should include and how it should be taught. Attempts to develop appropriate curriculum content for courses in public health and preventive medicine for both students and residents are now under way, much of the impetus coming from the Academies of Family Practice and Public Health (American Academy of Family Practice 1986).

One problem in having the relationship between social events and illness being accepted as valid information for medical students is the skepticism of these data expressed by our scientifically trained colleagues in medical schools. Part of the difficulty lay in the inability of previous psychosomatic theoreticians to construct scientifically plausible connections between psychosocial factors and disease pathogenesis. Now with the enormous advances in our understanding of the pervasive regulatory function of the brain on bodily processes, sophisticated hypotheses of disease pathogenesis incorporating psychosocial as well as biological factors are possible (Hendrie 1986). A course that incorporates information from the social sciences attached to a neurobiological framework is now more likely to be acceptable to both faculty and students.

However, rather than burden the poor harassed medical student with even more facts and additional courses on top of the existing material, what is required is the introduction of this material in a manner compatible with the overall philosophy of the medical school curriculum. This could involve a radical restructuring of the entire curriculum to reflect the quickly evolving new concepts of disease, as long advocated by Engel (1978, 1980). Along these lines Weiner (1988) described a four-year course in behavioral biology and medicine that could act as a cornerstone for a medical school curriculum. It is conceivable, however, that the teaching of "biopsychosocial" medicine could be incorporated into the existing disease state-oriented curriculum if the teaching (and clinical care) were more multidisciplinary than is currently the case.

Information on public health and social medicine would not by itself promote humane care by physicians. It would, however, provide a much broader and more balanced perspective for physicians who are likely to be involved in major decisions regarding the establishment of priorities for the utilization and distribution of health care resources in the future. In combination with the advances in knowledge in the neurobiological sciences, it also provides a scientific rationale for emphasizing the importance of the development of interpersonal and communicational skills in physicians.

Skills

During the course of medical school education, students are required to learn many technical skills in order to manage the increasingly sophisticated tools of their trade. This process is usually handled well, although instruction on how to interpret correctly the vast quantities of new data provided by this advanced technology is often deficient, as is the ability to analyze critically the clinical literature based upon these findings. Two crucial skills are often overlooked, however: the ability to communicate and the ability to acquire and access knowledge.

Amid the current debates and disagreements among medical educators about the most appropriate educational content and process for medical students, there is unanimity on one item: the necessity for the development of good communication skills by physicians. That this is not happening at present is also evident. "Given the necessity to communicate frequently and freely, I never cease to be amazed at how poorly the medical profession does it. . . . Instead of using the mother tongue, quite an elegant vehicle to transmit our thoughts in clear, relatively brief sentences, we obfuscate them in jargon and incomprehensible abbreviations. . . . Out with the mumblers and the scribblers! Clarity of speech and writing breed elevation of thought and Lord knows we need more of that." Thus Petersdorf (1986) sounds the clarion call for the development of communication skills in physicians. The requirement of good communication skills in physicians in order to elicit information, impart information, and provide support and encouragement to patients as well as to participate in the health education of the general public is obvious. Dr. Dickstein, in her chapter, reviews the current problems of the development of communication skills in medical students and discusses various solutions.

A major thrust of the GPEP report "Physicians for the Twenty-First Century" (1984) was to emphasize the necessity for physicians to acquire the learning skills necessary to keep abreast of the explosion of new scientific information. Its recommendations included encouraging independent learning skills, reducing scheduled time and lecture hours, using evaluative methods that emphasize the students' analytic skills rather than their ability to memorize, and the designation of one academic unit in medical schools to provide leadership in the application of informational services and computer technology to medical students and physicians. Clearly, even since this report was published in 1984, both the information explosion and the development of sophisticated computer technology to allow easy access to this information has continued apace. Almost every physician in the country has in his or her office a computer terminal. Medical schools and other privately funded organizations are busy manufacturing software which will provide to physicians through their terminals vast amounts of detailed information and in the near future provide consultative services about individual patients as well as allow laboratory data to be analyzed in a centralized facility. This easy access to the general practitioner of information and expertise could potentially revolutionize medical care, greatly expanding the ability of primary care physicians to care for patients with complicated illnesses in the community. This expanded information base, incidentally, will also be available to a large extent to the general public, leading to an even more knowledgeable and sophisticated patient population that is likely to demand more sharing of responsibilities for medical decisions. Some cable channels are already transmitting large quantities of medical information intended for the general public.

Yet little change has occurred in medical school curricula and evaluative methods, most of which still emphasize the acquisition of information and test memorized learning. The absurdity of basing the success or failure of medical students on their ability to recollect large amounts of information in testing situations of relative sensory isolation when for the rest of their lives they are likely to be bombarded with instant information and will be required to select only the most relevant items in order to practice properly is all too obvious.

Summary

Two major classes of events have led to a reconsideration of medical student education. The first is the explosion of knowledge in the social sciences and neurobiology, which not only correlates psychosocial events with health and illness but also provides a framework for understanding the mechanism whereby these events produce their effects. The second is the change in social climate with the advent of more sophisticated consumers who demand more openness and equality in interactions with physicians. These developments have focused interest again on doctors' interactions with patients and highlight the potential therapeutic value of good communications skills. The attitudes, knowledge, and skills for physicians which will be required to practice in this new environment have been discussed.

REFERENCES

American Academy of Family Practice (1986). *Newsletter,* reprint no. 269.
American Board of Internal Medicine, Subcommittee on Evaluation of Humanistic Qualities in the Internist (1983). *Annals of Internal Medicine* 99:720–724.
American College of Preventive Medicine (1987). Residency Training Manual for Preventive Medicine, developed by the Graduate Education Committee.

Bloom, B. (1976). *A Taxonomy of Educational Objectives*. New York: McKay.

Bulger, R. J. (1987). A dialogue with Hippocrates and Griff T. Ross, M. D. In *In Search of the Modern Hippocrates*. Bulger, R. J. (ed.), Iowa City: University of Iowa Press, 253.

Dighton, R. (1970). Cartoon (plate 90) in *Medicine and the Artist*, 3d ed. Carl, Z. (ed.), New York: Dover.

Engel, G. L. (1978). The biopsychosocial model and the education of health professionals. *Annals of New York Academy of Science* 310:169–181.

Engel, G. L. (1980). The clinical application of the biopsychosocial model. *American Journal of Psychiatry* 137:535–544.

GPEP Report (1984). Physicians for the twenty-first century. *Journal of Medical Education* 59:11.

Hendrie, H. C. (1986). The brain and the biopsychosocial approach to medicine. In *Neuroregulation of Autonomic, Endocrine and Immune Systems*. Frederickson, R. C. A., Hendrie, H. C., Hingtgen, J. N., and Aprison, M. H. (eds.), Boston: Martinus Nijhoff, 1–6.

Indiana University (1912). *Bulletin*, May 15, 1912, 44.

Lerner, M. (1975). *Saturday Review*, November 1.

Newsweek (1987). The revolution in medicine, January 26.

Petersdorf, R. G. (1986). Medical education for the future: A mandate for change. *Internist*, May–June, 17–20.

Schofield, J. R. (1984). New and Expanded Medical Schools, Mid-Century to the 1980s. Association of American Colleges, Washington, D.C., 294.

Starr, P. (1982). *The Social Transformation of American Medicine*. New York: Basic Books.

Stoeckle, J.D. (1987). *Encounters between Patients and Doctors*. Cambridge, Mass.: MIT Press, 3.

Weiner, H. (1988). A proposal for a curriculum in behavioral biology and medicine in medical schools. In *Experimental Foundations of Behavioral Medicine: Conditioning Approaches*. Ader, R., Weiner, H., and Bamm, A. (eds.), Hillsdale, N.J.: Lawrence Erlbaum Associates, 175–184.

White, K. L. (1988) The task of medicine. In *Dialogue at Wickenburg*. Henry J. Kaiser Family Foundation, Menlo Park, Calif., 52.

Part Two

Current Medical Education and the Development of Humaneness

The structure and functioning of the medical school is analyzed in this part with respect to its impact on the development of humanistic qualities in medical students and residents. In the first essay, Roger Bulger focuses on the need for medical schools to develop an integrated, schoolwide educational philosophy regarding what the characteristics or qualities of the ideal physician are and then on the need to construct a learning environment conducive to fostering the development of these exemplary characteristics. He observes that the model of patient care which medical students receive during their training tends to be fragmented and highly specialized, emphasizing seriously ill inpatients while deemphasizing continuity of care and less seriously ill outpatients where psychosocial issues may be especially prominent. The net result of this educational process is that medical students have little access to models of comprehensive and humane patient care, from either the faculty or the resident staff. Bulger also notes that there is an analogy between the faculty-student relationship and the doctor-patient relationship; how the faculty interacts with students may in turn affect how students interact with patients under their care.

The second essay, by Camille Lloyd and Ann Gateley, considers the educational process as it affects medical students and residents themselves. These authors detail how highly stressful medical education can be and document aspects of the medical education experience that may serve to adversely affect both the student/residents' own well-being and their subsequent approach to patient care. The essay complements Bulger's by amplifying specific aspects of the medical education system which impede the development of humaneness in medical trainees. It also anticipates part three by briefly introducing recent developments in educational programs that address the human needs and feelings of medical trainees and in turn prepare trainees to address the human needs and feelings of patients.

The Impact of the Educational System on the Development of the Modern Hippocrates

ROGER J. BULGER

The phrase "the modern Hippocrates" implies an operational goal for the educational system, an agreed-upon vision of professional and behavioral characteristics that are quintessential for the modern physician. It is safe to say that there is no such uniformly accepted portrait of the new physician as a young woman or young man; there are in fact all too few medical schools that have made a serious effort at defining in some detail the behavioral patterns they would determine to be essential to the excellent physician. Even fewer schools seem to have accepted the idea that the school's environment could be tailored to support the development of those characteristics deemed exemplary and desirable. Thus, it should not be surprising that all too often a school's environment in fact encourages the development of personal behaviors antithetical to those of the excellent physician. These observations probably derive from the basic fact that the influences of the behavioral sciences are unevenly expressed and embraced in medical schools across the land. Some apologists for the current situation might well argue that the ancient Hippocratic oath and the associated tradition of Western scientific medicine has produced a commonsense image of the kind of doctor we all want. They might further believe that at the heart of the entrepreneurial nature of their physician there needs to be a certain individualism and toughness so that the ideal paradigm should sail through all sorts of negative forces in the educational or any other environment to hone in unerringly on those behaviors known to be correct. The argument can be made that the educational environment really doesn't matter in the final product as long as the requisite academic excellence is required. It is difficult to prove, for example, that physicians graduated from a noncompetitive, supportive medical school are more sensitive, compassionate, and psychologically balanced than are those who completed a highly competitive, dog-eat-dog curriculum.

William May has illustrated the possible variations on the theme of physicianhood in *The Physician's Covenant,* wherein he describes the doctor as parent or fighter or technician or teacher or covenantor.[1] Clearly, in reality, the complex final human product will have varying percentages of each of these ingredients, and there should be no implication that the best goal is a physician who fits purely into just one of these molds. Another recent volume[2] brings together a number of views of modern physicianhood and culminates by attempting to translate those views into a modern oath of Hippocrates, which in turn delimits the behavioral playing field for the best of the modern healers.

A brief descriptive summary of such an ideal physician is as follows: competent, caring, communicative, committed to enhancing the health of the patient and to helping the patients help themselves, capable of handling pressure well and of facing calamitous situations in the lives of others with great equilibrium. Fitting these characteristics into the May classification, we would agree that there is little room for the authoritative, parenting mode. There is on the other hand room for the fighter against disease and suffering and the excellent technician who knows how to get things done when things need to be done. However, the underlying commitment or covenant provides the basis out of which the physician as teacher emerges, and the physician as teacher becomes the healer not only in the acute disease situation but also through aiding the patient to achieve a successful adjustment to chronic disease and by means of promoting health in the life of the individual person.

It is important at this point that the reader be made aware of some of my own biases about the effects of the educational process on the learner. The first bias is that the educational environment is important to the educational outcome; it does matter to the student how people, data, and resources are treated. My second bias is that what we do not know far exceeds what we do know and that a great deal of what we think we know will be shown to be incorrect in the years ahead; thus integrity and humility ought to be encouraged. My third bias is that the role model of the teacher is far more important than most teachers seem to appreciate and that the analogy between the student/teacher relationship and the patient/physician relationship is not lost upon students even if some faculty don't seem to appreciate it. With these biases in mind, let us proceed to some of the elements of modern medical education which may work against the development of our ideal physician.

Increasingly, schools of medicine seek to develop an overall, schoolwide educational philosophy, but it must be admitted that in many places the departmental imperative holds sway. That is, the functional educational philosophy experienced by students is that of the department in which they find themselves at any given time. Thus in one school it might be possible to find several philosophies in place, leading to an educational situation which on balance cannot be said to promote a consistent behavior on the part of the student.

It has long been pointed out that there is a problem inherent in the teaching and role-modeling area when the faculty are chosen for scientific achievements and technical skills primarily. They must be major achievers in the "publish or perish" environment, and they have therefore other factors claiming precedence over their teaching and service functions. That this has been so often identified as a problem makes it no less real as a factor in many schools.

In recent years, as the march of high technology seems to have gone forward at a redoubled pace, with much of it in the clinical departments of our medical schools, the faculty's clinical practice has generated tremendous resources. The dollars have become an enormous factor in the financing of the departments and indeed of the entire school. In the press of all that high technology and big business, it must be easy for modern academic subspecialists to forget the needs of individual students and their own function as caregivers in addition to technology purveyors.

Obviously, medical students have lived a life of enormous drive through high school and college in order to gain admission to medical school. In medical school, the pace of the work in the first two years continues to press students to place their own goals and objectives above those of others, the exact reverse of what is most desirable in a mature caregiver. The pressure to perform well remains high in medical school, where one is seldom rewarded for confessing ignorance; in a variety of settings, one learns that to get the highest grades, one is better off hazarding a guess. Clearly, an environmental pattern emerges which in fact encourages a kind of deceptive behavior, again contravening our objective of developing a physician of great integrity, constantly on the lookout for what is not known and willing to easily admit to not knowing, while at the same time moving to correct that deficiency. It isn't so bad not to know something important; but it is bad to remain ignorant for very long after one learns of one's ignorance of something important to know. These kinds of pressures make it seem counterproductive to spend extra time just to get to know a patient better or in assisting a colleague with a problem instead of beating him or her to answers to questions the professor might be asking at the next rounds. It always seems demeaning of the character of medical students when comments such as these are made about them. Such generalizations are of course necessarily inaccurate; the real situation is much more complex. The nature of the material to be learned and the life and death ethos place the learner in a position of great stress. Students must learn all the important material or be found wanting, guilty perhaps someday of contributing to someone's demise because of intellectual laziness. The knowledge is the key and the pursuit is never-ending; time spent on things other than acquiring this knowledge or applying it is somehow useless and provokes a sense of guilt in the learner. Family, friends, culture, sports, religion, politics, all are of secondary importance to the monarchy of medicine.

In recent years, a new dimension has been added to the aspiring student's environmental enemies. The financial facts of life seem to be that most students graduate from medical school in debt between fifty and one hundred thousand dollars. Not long ago, most financial analysts would have advised that such was a good financial position to be in assuming the graduate was healthy, because earning potential was so great. These days, however, when starting salaries for young physicians are quite limited and opportunities to go into any specialty one chose have long since vanished, the problem of severe debt has to be a highly threatening specter, one which could dramatically affect the approach of an otherwise well-intentioned physician.

The clinical years bring what one has thought of as science into the realm of the practical. Students often believe they have been taught basic science for the first two years and that now comes the practical part. Interestingly, the approach of most doctor of philosophy programs to the basic sciences is considerably different than that experienced by medical students. Still, it sometimes seems to the medical students that questions are raised ad nauseum in the first two years. Enter the world of certainty, where even the best of clinicians hang what they choose to remember of the basic sciences upon a clinical framework that makes sense of their current experience, that in and of itself helps the doctor to remember that vast latticework of clinical material leading to proper diagnosis and treatment. Forgotten too easily by clinicians are those studies in the basic sciences which make no clinical sense; those are the things they ignore and have selectively forgotten. When the newly emergent clinical student raises a question based on something learned last year but which falls in the "to be forgotten" category, the clinical professor directly or indirectly lets the student know how lightly he or she regards that particular fact and that particular question. It is hard to keep up the open questioning in the midst of the need to be so certain about so much, in an environment when so much is known that can lead to practical improvement for the sufferer. The best professors can do it much of the time, but all too many of us simply find it much more fun to pass on what we know and deemphasize our limitations.

One major objective of the education of the budding clinician is to gain proficiency in the handling of medical emergencies, to work ever more effectively against the press of time, to shorten oral presentations to the salient facts, to learn the essentials of clinical thinking in diagnosis and treatment. It is essential to become confident of one's ability to handle all common emergencies before one can become comfortable enough to really relax in the clinical situation such that the learning goes on most efficiently. In my experience, this occurs for most people in the first postgraduate year, for some exceptional students in the fourth year of medical school and for others in their second postgraduate year. Since the hospital is where the emergency situations occur in greatest number and where the greatest intensity of clinical experience with a wide array of cases may be found, it is not surprising that it is in the hospital that most of the education has been carried out. Clearly, this orientation leads to disease and case orientation rather than people emphases. Students get to know disease as it is manifested in people to whom they are exposed episodically; they do not get to know people in a longitudinal manner who experience disease and handle it in a variety of ways. So too, it may be argued, is it for the full-time, hospital-based, specialty-oriented faculty. It is hard in this pedagogical situation to keep promoting all those wonderful traits of the physician we described at the outset.

Lewis Thomas[3] describes the modern teaching hospital's environment as beautifully and succinctly as anyone has:

> . . . medicine is still stuck, for an unknowable period, with formidable problems beyond the reach of therapy or prevention. The technologies for making an accurate diagnosis have been spectacularly effective, and at the same time phenomenally complex and expensive. This new activity is beginning to consume so much of the time of the students and interns, and the resources of the hospital in which they do their work, that there is less and less time for the patient. Instead of the long, leisurely ceremony of history taking, and the equally long ritual of the complete physical examination, and then the long explanations of what has gone wrong and a candid forecast of what may lie ahead, the sick person perceives the hospital as an enormous whirring machine, with all the professionals—doctors, nurses, medical students, aides, and porters out in the corridors—at a dead run. Questionnaires, fed into computers along with items analyzing the patient's financial capacity to pay the bills, have replaced part of the history, and the CAT scan and Nuclear Magnetic Resonance machines are relied upon as more dependable than the physical examination.
>
> Everyone, even the visitors, seems pressed for time; there is never enough time; the whole place is over-worked to near collapse, out of breath, bracing for the next irremediable catastrophe—the knife wounds in the Emergency Ward, the flat lines on the electroencephalogram, the cardiac arrests, and always everywhere on every ward and in every room the dying. The old Hippocrates adage, "Art is long, Life is short," is speeded up to a blur.

In the clinical years in most schools, the format for learning is the graded responsibility model of the clinical team with students, junior residents, senior residents, and faculty member. This model is designed to work economically in the teaching hospital, where at every possible option the apparatus has traditionally been geared to adjust to the doctors' time and wishes. In recent years, however, the students' and doctors' time has become less important; the press of finances has shortened hospital stays and the incentives will continue to drive toward shortened times in hospital. The net result of that has been to play havoc with the traditional training programs, both for students and residents. It is economically sound practice to begin many work-ups in the outpatient department, with the patient entering the hospital only for essential tests or complex treatments that can't be done outside. Thus, students are confronting patients whose diagnosis has already been established and for whom the press of time before a major diagnostic or therapeutic intervention is so great that the student gets only the most truncated of exposures to "clinical material" which used to remain around long enough for intellectual digestion of the problem, process, and proposed treatment.

Although this extraordinarily deep pedagogical problem has been getting much discussion, very few schools have been able to change their approaches in order to amalgamate the in- and outpatient experiences for the students and residents. It is hard for professors of internal medicine to give up on such a tried and true tool as the graded responsibility model that has been so comfortably effective over the past sixty years. To persist with the current model, however, is in my view to minimize the educational opportunities of the students. Very few faculties realize that their curricular approaches can be negative, that their corporate decisions and practices can hurt their own students. Like most of the human race, faculty are unlikely to change their approach until something dramatic happens.

Interestingly, just this past year internal medicine residencies went begging which in the past have always been the object of the most intense competition among the most proficient of students. Why? There is no answer yet to this question, although we are getting rather glib answers in the face of no data. The most popular answers seem to be that the AIDS epidemic and the onslaught of the elderly has made internal medicine less appealing. Although some of this may be true, it may also be that the fragmented experience of the hospital-oriented internal medicine training is of diminishing interest to students. Students are certainly opting in large numbers for the procedure-oriented, high technology, acute-care-dominated diagnostic and therapeutic specialties. They seem not to be choosing the chronic care situation where the minimization of suffering is important, where little gains and improvements are the rule rather than the big dramatic cures. Possibly we don't select students who might likely find meaning caring for the chronically ill, and possibly we haven't found faculty who find such work exciting and stimulating and are able to transmit that enthusiasm to the students.

Melvin Konner, a professional anthropologist who went through medical school at age thirty-five, has written a book on medical education which deals primarily with the third year of medical school in which he describes his reactions to the various specialties as he experiences them.[4] It should be noted that Konner decided against an internship and returned to the anthropology classroom, and his book has the character of the typical study of a strange, archaic culture by a visiting anthropologist; it is a book, nonetheless, of considerable interest. Konner describes a clinical teaching year seemingly characterized by an almost total absence of senior faculty physicians; the students are left solely with the interns and residents for guidance. Lewis Thomas, in his review of Konner's book, questions (as my own experience makes me do) the validity of the implication that the faculty are invisible; at the same time, he recognizes the forces and realities that have diminished the role-modeling capacity of the senior faculty:

> Everyone is too busy, urgently doing something else, and there is no longer enough time for the old meditative, speculative ward rounds or the amiable conversations at the bedside. The house staff, all of them—interns, residents, junior fellows in for the year on NIH training fellowships—are careening through the corridors on their way to the latest "code" (the euphemism for the nearly dead or the newly dead, who too often turn out to be, in the end, the same), or deciphering computer messages from the diagnostic laboratories, or drawing blood and injecting fluids, or admitting in a rush the newest patient. The professors are elsewhere, trying to allocate their time between writing out their research requests (someone has estimted that 30 percent of a medical school faculty's waking hours must be spent composing grant applications), doing or at least supervising research in their laboratories, seeing their own patients. . . .

Clearly, to the extent that Konner and Thomas accurately describe hospital-based clinical teaching, there is much to correct and reorient if we wish to develop a curriculum conducive to the emergence of the new physician.

It is essential to mention the malpractice situation when discussing the pedogogy of clinical medicine these days. It is hard to underestimate the pervasive psychological effect of the malpractice threat within the schools. Just as it is often disconcerting to reflect on how dominant is the theme of earning and collecting money in the meetings of clinical departmental chiefs, it is equally disconcerting to reflect upon the frequency with which faculty interject the threat of malpractice into their teaching. Without attempting to take a position on the questions of law involved, I believe it is safe to assert that the overall impact of the malpractice situation is to drive the doctor-patient relationship toward a contract situation and away from a covenantal mode; and therein is a stake driven between the aspiring student and achievement of the status of the modern Hippocrates we described earlier.

Money is striking at the heart of the profession in many ways, overt and subtle. The pro-competitive scene has struck health care with a vengeance, and academic doctors are nothing if not great competitors. The entrepreneurial nature of successful clinical chairpersons and the sheer magnitude of the financial stakes have led many departments in many schools to be more concerned with money and efficiency for the sake of profit than used to be the case. These factors are not necessarily as parochial or selfish as they at first may seem to the outsider, because to a large extent the behavior of academicians has come to be governed by the need to survive in the marketplace. The inexorable super-specialization of medicine has led to departmentally focused resident and fellow educational programs usually funded through departmental efforts and often subliminally taking a kind of existential preference in the faculty's mind to medical student teaching. The latter phenomenon once again teaches the student that he or she is least important, and that is not the best example or model for placing the patient (truly the most vulnerable person in the chain) highest on the priority list. Specialization tends to minimize considerations of the total life situation of the patient, which is after all what the mature physician must deal with.

At still another level, most medical schools have been unsuccessful at providing a model multispecialty group practice exemplifying the best of such practices in the present day. The implication here is that the medical school faculty has the obligation to demonstrate excellence in its health care delivery efforts; in most instances, the multispecialty nature of the faculty should position them to organize model comprehensive care units. In failing to be imaginative and creative in their corporate health care efforts, the schools' faculties often subject their patients to less than optimal situations from a service and humane point of view—also a negative example for the students.

In sum, medical school clinical departments are often big, high technology businesses, upon which the welfare of the teaching hospital depends, doing many different things very well but not optimally preparing students for the world they must face. Even the most committed and articulate voice arguing against the so-called medical-industrial complex speaks through a medical-scientific journal enjoying a multimillion-dollar advertising bonanza, a paradox not lost on most observers (including our aspiring young Hippocrates, who notes the juxtaposition of the glossy full-page ads with the high science of the journal articles).

Finally, although there has been a lot of talking over the years and although some institutions may have taken some steps in the right direction, medical educators will have to confess that there is all too little interprofessional education. The need is for better contact and communication with dentists, pharmacists, allied health personnel; and especially important with regard to the hospital environment are nurses. The nurses have become the human glue holding the teaching (or any other) hospital together, and it is absolutely essential from the patients' perspective to develop superior teamwork and unity among the various health team members if there is to be any significant hope of achieving the goal of humane care of the highest technical quality.

Against this litany of negative pedagogical influences, can we discover any saving graces? Aren't we doing something right? Of course, we are doing things right; to be perfectly honest, there is no medical education I would prefer to that available in the United States. Furthermore, there are many thoughtful educators who do understand the social forces acting on the profession and who are thinking about better ways of educating their students to the essential humanity of the healer. Just as there is a list of forces working against the development of the modern Hippocrates, there is another list of forces which will work to facilitate the new healing paradigm.

The first of these new and positive influences is what I perceive to be an emerging sense of the unity of intellectual efforts. We find the evidence all around us. C. P. Snow's division of the intellectual world into the artistic and the scientific is being challenged. Creativity is seen as the same process whether it takes place in a poet or a theoretical physicist. Physicists, considering the universe and its origin and future, have public dialogues which remind the intelligent citizen of theologians; Teilhard de Chardin and process theologians seem to be saying that the search for new understanding in nature is the search for God. Recent advances in the study of the brain, its bicameral nature, its biochemistry, and its pharmacology have in effect caused a revolution in our conceptions about ourselves with important implications for our own health, implications we are only just beginning to understand in a pragmatic sense.

One of the more startling impacts of the neurochemical revolution is the realization that the literally thousands of known chemicals operative in our brains, including the endorphins, constitute a veritable pharmacy; increasingly, both doctors and patients appreciate the power of that pharmacy and the importance of learning how to use it properly. Thus, even the most biochemically oriented of young physicians in training can understand how the doctor's words and affect can positively or negatively influence the patient's well-being through chemical reactions in the brain. It is, I believe, this central phenomenon which is serving to bring together the scientific, biomedical model and the holistic approaches to health. There is at least a common ground whereon some new understandings can emerge.

Linguist Walter Ong says of the modern era that it is the age of the new orality, an age wherein the written word no longer predominates and children grow up with earphones listening to rock stars who lead through their use of their voices. This is the sort of world in which a new healer could emerge, more adept than his or her predecessors in the uses of the presence, the voice, or the word in creating a therapeutic environment, in which patients are aided in efforts to use their own powers in addition to direct interventions such as surgery or chemotherapy.[2]

The so-called informed consent movement has slipped onto the clinical stage, influencing dramatically the nature of the doctor-patient interaction and giving it a shape which should in turn offer new opportunities for the emerging physician. It is uncertain how clearly our faculties understand what has emerged from the informed consent doctrine. Entering our culture through the clinical investigation window in the early 1960s, the need for the patient to be adequately informed has spread from the clinical investigation world to the everyday world of clinical practice, so that it is the legal responsibility of the physician to ensure that the patient fully understands the risks of the various diagnostic or therapeutic options to be utilized; the patient has become an important decision-maker in determining his or her own care. Although many physicians and patients still operate under and prefer the authoritarian, paternalistic mode with the doctor as the sole decision-maker, it seems clear that our society is moving rapidly to one wherein the patient and the family are the decision-makers as much as is possible and the physician is the junior partner in that regard and must relate differently to the patient than in the past. With the growing effectiveness of our technology and with the physician as the purveyor of that technology, there is a new opening and plenty of room for the sensitive physician to establish a patient relationship in a therapeutic manner.

The future necessitates an educational present for which many of our faculties are ill-prepared. As they deal with the computer age, the imaging age, the technological imperative, our schools must also deal with the exploding fields of the biobehavioral sciences—and most current medical school faculty members (especially the older, established academic leaders) just don't give much currency to the latter. For example, there is no doubt that the placebo effect is real; there can also be no doubt that almost no consideration is given such an important subject in the current medical curriculum. Many of our best ethicists tell us that we shouldn't use placebos because their use is basically a deception of the patient; scientists and biomedically oriented clinicians often feel that getting the benefits of the placebo effect is cheating and shouldn't "count," because it isn't really treating the molecular defect with an externally administered agent. Still, many of holistic medicine's approaches and other, perhaps more accepted behaviors and treatments may well turn out to be only placebo effect. Now we think or at least can envision that placebos and other things such as kind words, sympathy, and trust may release chemicals from our own intra-cranial pharmacy which may in fact work on the disease or its symptoms at the molecular level. If the doctor can learn how to more reliably tap the patient's own therapeutic resources, a new dimension of scientific healing should be open for fuller exploitation.

In fact, we may be seeing evidence now that a new physician is emerging in the modern Western democracies, especially in the United States and Canada, where the patient is moving rapidly into the driver's seat with relation to his or her own care. More young doctors are learning from the social sciences and even the arts during their medical educations. Artists, whose business it is to communicate with other human beings, are teaching medical students how to listen, how to look and to see, how to feel what someone else is trying to communicate to them; these skills represent an essence of physicianhood that threatened to become vestigial in recent decades.

As communication skills and interviewing techniques become more obviously important in the overall scheme of things, these subjects have in some instances received an approach equal to the approach to physiology, for example. Thus, some years back, I can remember an internist friend cum expert on interviewing telling medical students that an emotionally neutral approach was the only way to get scientifically valid historical data; thus, a supportive, friendly demeanor implying sympathy, empathy, and friendship was unsatisfactory. I could see Hippocrates rolling over in the Elysian fields with colic at this development. A poet or a playwright might be more enlightening for some students in the long run.

Certainly, there is no clear path to a better future and a new physician paradigm. We have much to learn. We have many bright people trying to learn as they are trying to interpret the world around them. The best people know that we remain steeped in ignorance, and it may be just as well that there is now no dominant force in this chaotic picture of health care. By refocusing on competence, caring, communication, and community, we might well reinvigorate our staggering sense of educational direction. There are positive signs in that direction, but only an historian sometime in the future will know and understand. As participants in the change and the turmoil, we never can be sure we know anything significant about it.

Paradoxically, if medicine loses some of its lofty financial and social status, it might turn out that those best suited to meet the care needs of our society will continue to seek out places in the profession and to gain entry to our schools. In England, despite physician overcrowding there is no feeling of a loss in quality or commitment among the students. In our case, a smaller, tighter, more committed army of healers might emerge side by side with the scientist-technicians required to manage our extraordinary diagnostic and therapeutic interventions.

In the end, all persons are in charge of their own educations. We must trust that bright, well-educated physicians in training will take the best from our offerings and will incorporate them to their best educational advantage. No new Hippocratic paradigm will emerge without the students willing that it should be so.

REFERENCES

1. May, William F. *The Physician's Covenant—Images of the Healer in Medical Ethics.* Westminster Press, Philadelphia, 1983.

2. Bulger, R. J. *In Search of the Modern Hippocrates.* University of Iowa Press, Iowa City, 1987.

3. Thomas, Lewis. "What Doctors Don't Know." *New York Review of Books,* September 24, 1987, 6–10.

4. Konner, Melvin. *Becoming a Doctor: A Journey of Initiation in Medical School.* Viking, New York, 1987.

SEVEN

Facilitating Humaneness in Medical Students and Residents

CAMILLE LLOYD AND ANN GATELEY

Throughout history the goal of medical education has been to select and train humane physicians. For twenty-five centuries the Hippocratic oath has served as the standard of those human qualities to which the nascent physician should aspire. Indeed, the ancient Hippocratic manuscripts clearly indicate that the medical profession exists to benefit human life (Osler 1921). The past several decades, however, have witnessed a growing debate as to whether medicine is a profession more of the sciences or of the healing arts. Spectacular technological progress has occurred, perhaps obscuring medicine as art. Some charge that medical educators have abandoned teaching communication and interpersonal skills in favor of teaching more technical skills, such as the interpretation of nuclear magnetic resonance imaging.

Most likely both laymen and physicians alike would agree that the display of concerned, empathic attention is still the sine qua non of the doctor-patient relationship. However, the profession appears to be assailed from within and from without by forces which mitigate against the maintenance of a compassionate and humane approach to patient care. Is this indeed true? And, if so, why?

Evidence from a number of sources indicates that there is indeed good reason for concern about the deterioration of the interpersonal aspects of patient care. Many older clinicians, for example, have noted the increasingly common habit of depersonalizing patients. This depersonalization takes the form of referring to patients as "cases"; of using multiple depreciating epitaphs including "gomer" and "turkey"; and so forth. There have also been multiple documentations that both house officers and attending physicians have poor interviewing styles. Platt and McMath (1979) observed more than three hundred clinical interviews and found that physicians previously judged as competent primary clinicians were actually impeding the establishment of rapport and the collection of an accurate data base from their patients. Duffy et al. (1980) observed sixty clinic visits and concluded that clinicians' interpersonal skills were exceedingly under-developed. Defective skills lay in the area of "recognizing the patient is a person with an illness and specific coping capacity that he and his family may use to deal with the illness." Beckman and Frankel (1984) further documented deficits in a study which revealed that the medical interview, previously thought of as the sacrosanct opportunity to forge a rapport with one's patient and to elicit present and potential medical problems, was being tightly controlled by the majority of physicians observed. Such a highly controlled interviewing style served to cut off patients before they were able to fully express their concerns, limited the rapport developed and the amount of useful information obtained, and contributed to the "by the way" phenomenon where the patient finally expresses his or her major concern as the physician is heading out the door. Deterioration of a quality doctor/patient relationship is also suggested by the rapid escalation in the number of malpractice suits filed and in the consequent rise in the cost of medical malpractice insurance.

Schwartz and Wiggins (1985) have discussed the disenchantment of consumers of health care who, while satisfied with the technical competence and expertise of their physicians, have become increasingly dissatisfied with the human element of their care. Schwartz and Wiggins noted that while there has been a growing feeling that the technical quality of medical care is improving rapidly, physician skills in careful listening, empathic respond-ing, and communicating medical findings and treatment options to patients have been deteriorating. The public's great concern with maintaining a quality doctor/patient relationship is evident in the ongoing attention de-voted to the topic in the popular literature (see *Psychology Today*, November 1986, pages 22–26, and *Newsweek*, January 26, 1987, pages 57–59).

In addition to documenting defective interviewing styles and to the growing disenchantment on the part of patients with the human aspects of their medical care, the emergence of judgmental attitudes toward certain patient groups has also made medical educators fearful that the human aspect of medicine is being poorly taught. The burgeoning number of AIDS cases in recent years presents a major challenge for medical edu-cators. Kelly et al. (1987) investigated whether or not medical students were developing negative attitudes toward AIDS patients. His studies revealed that unexpectedly harsh, stigmatizing attitudes were present in a majority of students tested. Prejudice against AIDS patients will undoubtedly ad-versely affect a humanistic approach to this growing segment of the popu-lation. There have also been many instances where medical students and residents have refused to care for AIDS patients (Whalen 1987). Such a stance was previously rare; the history of medicine is replete with stories of physicians and nurses who submitted themselves to extremely hazardous conditions in order to care for their patients.

What has led to the decline of humaneness in the care of patients? In seeking to answer this question one might first ask whether the people selected for medical education and training are lacking in those basic qualities which allow an empathic response to patients? Are the students admitted to medical training today any different from those admitted previously? There is some indication that there are differences in the current medical student population. In the past, competition for medical school admission was keen, culminating in the highest number of applications in the early 1970s. In recent years, there has been a dramatic drop in applicants so that there are now less than two applicants for every medical school position available. There is also a trend toward lower MCAT scores and overall GPAs in current applicants. There are also more women and minority applicants. There is less stigma for the older student and for the student who has had a previous profession. Are these changes bad? Do they predispose to a student body that is less compassionate? Probably not; in fact, it has been argued that the admission of women, socialized to possess nurturing qualities, and the admission of students with greater life experiences would in fact favorably influence the humane aspects of medical care.

One may then ask whether the premedical school experience may alter or select individuals who are narrow, rigid, less compassionate? Certainly there are heavy emphases on rigorous science courses in the premedical curriculum. These requirements encourage applicants to acquire more hours and major in the life sciences. It is difficult, however, to ascertain whether today's applicants are more narrow than those of previous years. Furthermore, the British model of medical education telescopes eight years into six; applicants are solicited during their high school years and encounter a curriculum replete with scientific subjects for two or three years before entering clinics for the last three years. This truncated system has been examined many times, and it appears to turn out compassionate as well as competent clinicians (Mellinkoff 1987). While it may be premature to rule out the premedical experience and the selection process of medical school as partial contributors to the decline in the humane attributes of today's physicians, it would seem that something is occurring in the medical education system itself which fails to encourage or even actively inhibits the development of a humane approach to patient care.

Indeed, a number of factors in the medical educational system could mitigate against the development of patient-oriented physicians. To identify these factors, one can begin by assembling what is known about the process of the present medical educational system and by what is known about the impact of this system on the medical student and resident. The substantial literature on stress in medical school (Rosenberg 1971; Boyle and Coombs 1971; Coburn and Jovaisas 1975; Edwards and Zimet 1976;

Lloyd and Gartrell 1983) indicates that the medical student is exposed to a wide variety of stressors and that the intensity of this stress is relatively high, exceeding that of other health professional students (Bjorksten et al. 1983). In examining specific sources of stress, almost all studies implicate information overload as a major problem. While the knowledge base of medicine has been escalating rapidly since the Flexner model of medical education was introduced in 1910, the time allotted medical students to acquire and master the relevant basic science base of medicine has not shown any corresponding increase; students are still expected to acquire this knowledge within the first two years of medical school. The amount of information that a student can assimilate in two preclinical years cannot escalate forever; to ignore the student's limitation in this regard is to model inhumane expectations. Either educators must make a greater effort to set priorities regarding the information that students are required to learn or the time available to the student to master the scientific base of medicine will have to be lengthened.

The vast information to be learned in the preclinical years and the rapid pace at which this learning must occur prove beyond the grasp of some medical students. Rarely do those students who fall behind receive specialized opportunities to learn at their own pace. Although it is well known that rates of learning vary across individuals, current medical education programs require all students to master the material at the same rate. In the typical undergradaute setting, a student has many more options regarding the pace at which he or she chooses to proceed, since the number of semester hours taken is flexible. Hence, the persistent rigidity of requiring that an ever-growing body of knowledge be assimilated at a similar pace by everyone seems less than optimally humane.

Since students are now required to learn more rapidly and to learn more material, there is also less time available for meeting personal needs. Indeed, empirical studies consistently document that the lack of time for recreation and for development of friendships and family relationships is a second major source of stress for the student (Lloyd and Gartrell 1983). A medical school models a less than humane environment to the extent that it fails to acknowledge that students are human beings with very real social and recreational needs.

The inflexibility of the curriculum in most medical schools may detract from the humanistic milieu of the medical school in additional ways. It is not uncommon, for example, for a few students in every medical school class to suffer the death of a parent or sibling during the first or second year of medical school. Since the pace of the material presented is so rapid, the student who must miss one or two weeks of school to return home to attend the funeral or assist the family frequently falls so far behind that it is not possible to catch up on the academic requirements and resume studies for the year. The inflexibility of the curriculum and/or the unwillingness of course or school administrators to assist the student in establishing an alternate work or test schedule may result in the student's loss of the entire year. The consequences of such a situation are certainly not insubstantial; to the student already facing acute grief and feelings of loss, the additional loss of a structured setting and purpose for the remainder of the year, accompanied by the loss of a supportive network of class friends and the additional burden of financing another year of undergraduate medical education, can be psychologically detrimental. At times, therefore, the apparent inflexibility of curriculums or of medical school administrators to such a difficult personal situation of the student serves to model only inflexibility in response to human needs.

Another example of how a medical school environment may be antithetical to the development of humane interpersonal attitudes occurs when medical school administrators are rigidly prohibitive of transfers between institutions. In any medical school class, there will be a few students whose spouse will be required to relocate to another city because of job or educational requirements. The typical response of medical schools has been to prohibit or strongly discourage transfers during the four years of medical school. Dual career marriages or relationships are becoming more and more commonplace in today's society, yet little has been done in the society as a whole or in medical institutions to accommodate this situation. Medical education also takes place typically during the early adult years when individuals are appropriately concerned with establishing intimate and committed relationships. Consequently, there will be students whose educational requirements conflict strongly with their desire to be responsive to the needs of a spouse or partner whose own situation requires a relocation. Is it not possible for our medical schools to adopt at least a somewhat more flexible policy with respect to student transfers in order to accommodate these very real human dilemmas? The prohibition against student transfers was probably more reasonable when the traditional medical student was a man with a nonworking wife. But in today's society with dual career couples and with an increased number of women students, such inflexible rules seem only to model a failure to appreciate changing societal conditions and a nonresponsiveness to the personal and human needs of the students.

Not only does the curriculum of most medical schools result in a structure with minimum flexibility; the large impersonal nature of much of the teaching of the first two years often results in a feeling of dehumanization among the students. The rapid escalation of recent years in the number of medical students educated has resulted in large classes. Because the classes are large and everyone is desperately busy, "foxhole comradery" is less well developed. Many students do not know many of their classmates by name. Many can count the number of their friends on their hands. Small subgroups develop, but there appears to be a larger sense of overall isolation. Additionally, the large size of the class and the excessive amount of work seem to isolate the students from their professors as well. In an empirical study, Edwards and Zimet (1976) reported that almost half of the students in their survey reported that feelings of dehumanization were of major concern to them. The feelings of dehumanization were attributed to the experience of being an anonymous face in a crowded lecture hall and to being subjected to taxing academic demands where memorization and test-taking gamesmanship take precedence over individual initiative and mastery of important material. Feelings of dehumanization were also attributed to the dissonance students experience as a result of a curriculum that emphasizes the promotion of health and concern for the sick but fails to address the human needs of the students.

The lack of significant interaction with faculty during the preclinical years of medical school can also create the belief that teaching of students is a low priority in the medical school setting. Larger classes have brought increased teaching demands, and faculty have less time available for intensive interaction with students. The joy of teaching is diluted when the number of students becomes overwhelming.

In addition to a lack of significant interaction with medical faculty, students are also isolated from patient contact. Patients seem remote, unreachable, mysterious. Students often have little contact with patients until late in their second year. Does such a practice inadvertently convey the message that medicine is more about basic science knowledge than it is about serving people? One of the most common complaints of students in their preclinical years is the apparent lack of relevance of much of their learning to actual patient care (Moore-West et al. 1986). Such complaints reflect students' frustration with being isolated from patients and with the presentation of scientific material divorced from its relevance to the care of patients.

Most medical students look forward to their patient care years with a combination of eager anticipation and anxiety. During the third and fourth years, medical students finally get to care for patients. Because of recent radical changes in health care economics, however, patients admitted to teaching hospitals are fewer and considerably sicker than previously. Additionally, these patients have often been fully evaluated and followed in outpatient settings until hospitalization was inevitable. Such a situation deprives the student of seeing patients in their early stages of illness and of understanding the many factors which come into play in making diagnoses. Therefore the student's intervention is shifted away from the subtle beginnings of illness and the need for skillful elicitation of symptoms from patients, toward care of patients in their final stages of illness. The economic push to shorten hospital stays also means that the student may interact with the patient only during a major diagnostic or therapeutic intervention and has little time to develop a relationship with the patient, to understand the contribution of lifestyle factors to the development of the illness, to understand the impact of the illness on the patient, or to follow the outcome of the intervention.

Unfortunately, there is also little opportunity for students to learn in outpatient settings; it is not deemed to be time efficient. Students thus are deprived of developing an ongoing relationship with the patient. Consequently, they may be denied the experiences of learning how a physician can assist the patient in developing health-promoting behaviors, of learning how the physician can become an important patient educator, of learning how the physician can become an important confidant.

Because students learn by example, one can also ask about the student's clinical experiences with residents and attending physicians. To what extent are students themselves treated humanely by these senior physicians? To what extent do these residents and senior clinicians exemplify compassionate and interpersonally sensitive interactions with their patients? A recent report by Rosenberg and Silver (1984) indicates that, while most medical school administrators are oblivious to the problem, students report a significant exposure to episodes of verbal abuse and humiliation. While the majority of clinical teachers do an admirable job and interact respectfully with their students, the existence of a minority of individuals who justify their abusive actions as necessary for improved teaching does much to undermine the students' trust in the entire faculty. This is particularly the case when the offending clinician is a respected senior member of the faculty. Self-reports of physicians or physicians-in-training who perceived themselves to be the recipient of such abuse reveal that it resulted in their feeling angry and resentful; rendered them more nervous, less confident, and more emotionally constricted; and adversely affected their morale, motivation, and ability to learn (Rosenberg and Silver 1984).

Medical school faculty are experiencing increasing pressures themselves, pressures which compete with their desire to provide quality teaching and quality patient care. Faculty are increasingly preoccupied with obtaining research funding and with research productivity (Beeson 1987). Teaching skills are often undervalued; teaching duties within a department are often relegated to the younger and less experienced faculty and viewed as a necessary evil that will subsequently be handed down to new faculty as they are recruited. Indeed, the emphasis on research productivity rather than quality of clinical teaching that emerges in promotion and tenure decisions does not go unnoticed by medical school faculty (Petersdorf 1986). Students are also perceptive of medical school and departmental priorities.

Muller (1984) also observed these pressures on medical faculty. He commented that while many faculty were dedicated to the importance of the teacher/student relationship in medical education, the lack of institutional recognition for dedication to the educational mission interferes with their ability and willingness to make this crucial relationship a reality. He argued that impediments to change are systemic and institutional rather than personal.

Escalating financial pressures in medical schools are also resulting in increasing pressures on faculty to generate considerable income through the provision of clinical services. Senior faculty and administrators are increasingly becoming business executives focused on bed occupancy, collection of professional fees, etc. (Beeson 1987). Such activities take them away from patients' bedsides and away from the students eager to view senior clinicians in practice. Current pressures on medical school faculty appear to create a situation in which the faculty models self-promotion of their own research careers and an excessive concern with finances; the value of service to either the patient or the student is deemphasized.

Residents are also under the pressures of an increasingly sophisticated health care system. McCue (1985) posited that residency training has become more stressful over time because of the increasing factual knowledge base of medicine, the greater fear of malpractice suits, the larger number of hospitalizations of the elderly and chronically ill patients with more complex medical histories, and the greater amounts of time spent in clinical responsibilities, coordination of consultants, dictation of complicated discharge summaries, and scheduling of procedures. With such demanding responsibilities, residents face a severe shortage of time to teach students. They also face a shortage of time to devote to their learning, and hence often feel as though their own training needs take a distant second place to everyday clinical demands.

McCue (1985) also has enumerated many of the very stressful aspects of medical internship. Among the stressors he identified are the assumption of greater responsibility for patient care decisions, fear of inadequate performance, severe time pressures, and sleep deprivation. In addition to the stress directly associated with medical duties, interns often face new responsibilities of marriage and parenthood, financial pressures from accumulating debts, and the need to replace the friendships and emotional support of medical school. McCue also notes that the extreme time demands of residency (usually in excess of eighty hours a week) result in the melding of work and social relationships so that a strong potential is created for the development of narrow, culturally isolated physicians who do not appreciate the importance of citizenship and community activities. The extreme concentration of energy on vocational development inevitably detracts from energy available for personal development that should occur during the young adult years. In sum, the time pressures of internship and to a lesser extent of remaining residency years can approach such an extreme that they are antithetical to the development of a humanistically oriented physician. It is inconsistent to teach that we need physicians who are broadly trained in the social sciences and humanities and then to subject these same individuals to such severe time pressures that involvement in these activities is virtually precluded. It is dissonant also to teach residents the value to their patients of proper sleep, eating habits, and stress management and then to require of the interns and residents themselves behavior which is antithetical to their own well-being.

Only very recently has the issue of resident working hours been given more than lip service, as the New York State Health Department seeks to develop recommendations for limiting the number of hours house staff can work in a week (Glickman 1988; Petersdorf 1988). Indeed, it seems quite telling that it took a specific strong catalyst, the death of a patient, to finally obtain action with respect to excessive work hours. Additionally, one may note that attention seems to have been mobilized chiefly by issues of quality patient care rather than by valid issues of concern for the house staff. Equally noteworthy is that such changes were not born out of forces within the medical profession but rather such movement necessitated input from the courts and legal system as well.

In addition to commenting on these aspects of the medical education and training environment that may be antithetical to the development of humane attributes in students and residents, it may also be helpful to review the empirical literature regarding what is known about the impact of the medical education system on the student or resident. A variety of studies are available, including those which assess the impact of medical school on the student's health and lifestyle and those which assess the psychological consequences of the educational experience. Unfortunately, evidence from both of these research areas suggests some detrimental effects of the medical education process on the lifestyle and well-being of the student.

Kay et al. (1980) observed that 48 percent of freshmen and 68 percent of juniors reported that their attendance at one midwestern medical school was detrimental to their health. Huebner et al. (1981) concluded on the basis of interviews that time pressures compromised proper eating, sleeping, exercising, and relaxing in medical students. Wolf and Kisling (1984) documented a decrease in physical activity in freshmen and a decrease in time spent in recreational activities such as reading for pleasure, visiting with friends, etc. They also reported a decrease in the amount of sleep that students obtained and reported that very few students maintained a balanced diet. Perceived general health, both physical and psychological, was reported to decrease significantly over the course of the first year, with the most pronounced decrease relating to psychological or emotional health. In yet another survey, Green and Miyai (1986) reported that the majority of senior medical students exercised less than they had prior to medical school and also participated less in extracurricular activities. On other measures, however, there were indications that students increased the use of seat belts, decreased their intake of fatty foods, and felt that they had more friends and a better relationship with their parents than they had prior to medical school. The more positive results of this study may partially reflect the difference between sampling freshmen who are inundated by academic and adjustment demands and seniors whose demands have diminished. Clark and Rieker (1986) asked medical students to evaluate the impact of their graduate training on their relationships with spouses, lovers, roommates, family members, and friends; a majority of both men and women indicated that the stress of professional training had resulted in strained relationships, and a greater proportion of women than men stated that their primary relationship had ended during their training.

Possibly suggestive of a detrimental effect of medical education on the psychological well-being of medical students is an accumulating body of evidence suggesting (1) an increase in emotional distress during medical training (Davies et al. 1968; Lloyd and Gartrell 1981; Alagna and Morokoff 1986), (2) an increased suicide rate for women medical students (Pepitone-Areola-Rockwell et al. 1981), and (3) a fairly high prevalence of psychological symptoms (Lloyd and Gartrell 1984; Vitaliano et al. 1984) and disorder (Saslow 1956; Pitts et al. 1961; Hunter et al. 1961). Indeed, interview studies of medical students have provided estimates of the number of students identified as psychiatrically ill which range from 15 percent (Pitts et al. 1961) to 18 percent (Hunter et al. 1961) to 26 percent (Saslow 1956). A recent study using strict diagnostic criteria in interviews with students reported a prevalence rate of major depression of 12 percent during the first two years of medical school. The lifetime prevalence of major depression among medical students represented a statistically significant elevation from that found in 18- to 24-year-old general population controls. Taken together these studies suggest an elevated level of psychiatric symptomatology and disorder in medical students. However, these findings cannot unequivocally point to a detrimental impact of medical training on the student, since the possibility remains that such impairment may be due to the preexisting personality problems of the student (Vaillant et al. 1972; Bojar 1961; Roeske 1981). An unequivocal interpretation of such findings is also precluded since there is some evidence that students exposed to the rigors of law school show comparable or even greater symptom levels than those reported by medical students (Shanfield and Benjamin 1984; Kellner et al. 1986).

There are also a few studies which address how the medical school experience affects students' humanitarian qualities and their attitudes toward patients. Results suggest that medical students' cynicism increases and their idealism and humanitarianism decrease over the course of their medical training (Eron 1955; Becker and Geer 1958). Still, the number and breadth of such studies are quite limited, and little is known about what aspects of the educational experience underlie this apparent deterioration in humanitarianism.

While attention has been focused on the impact of medical training on students rather than residents, there is a small but growing empirical literature on the impact of internship and residency on the psychological well-being of the medical trainee. Literature on the effects of sleep deprivation in interns suggests that it is associated with depression, irritability, depersonalization, inappropriate affect, oversensitivity to criticism, and difficulties in thinking and recent memory (Friedman et al. 1973). The depression-evoking effect of residency training is becoming increasingly evident as research findings accumulate. Valko and Clayton (1975) reported in a retrospective survey that 30 percent of male interns were depressed and 18 percent had suicidal thoughts and a plan for committing suicide. Ford (1983) reported results of a questionnaire survey indicating that approximately one-third of the respondents had an episode of severe psychological distress, chiefly depression, during the internship year. Ford and Wentz (1984) reported that 40 percent of the interns felt that they had been clinically depressed during the year, and 15 percent actually met diagnostic criteria for a major depression. Clark et al. (1984) reported that a study of interns in medicine, surgery, pediatrics, and obstetrics and gynecology revealed that 27 percent developed a depressive syndrome during the first six months of the internship year. Reuben (1985) found a prevalence of depressive symptoms in 29 percent of medical interns and 21 percent of all house officers. Hsu and Marshall (1987), using the Center for Epidemiological Studies Depression Scale in a large-scale study of interns, residents, and fellows in Canada, reported that 26 percent of all male interns, 40 percent of all female interns, and 30 percent of the combined intern group showed some degree of depression. Examining the entire house staff group, 23 percent had some degree of depression. A recent study of interns in England by Firth-Cozens (1987) reported an estimated prevalence of emotional disturbance in 50 percent of the sample, with 28 percent showing evidence of depression. These studies taken together demonstrate the depressogenic effect of the internship year. In sum, self-reported depression in interns ranged from 29 percent to 40 percent, and the application of more stringent diagnostic criteria suggested that between 15 percent and 27 percent of interns develop a depressive disorder. These figures reflect a substantial inflation over what would be expected in age-matched general population or university student controls.

In addition to depression, Small (1981) described house officer's stress syndrome as consisting of seven features: episodic cognitive impairment, chronic anger, pervasive cynicism, family discord, depression, suicidal ideation and suicide, and substance abuse. He believed the first four features occurred in nearly all house officers.

Studies of mood changes in internal medicine interns demonstrated an increase in anger/hostility (Ford and Wentz 1984; Uliana et al. 1984) and levels of fatigue, depression, and defeat (Girard et al. 1986). When assimilated, therefore, the evidence is fairly convincing regarding the negative impact of the internship year on the intern's psychological health. There is some reason to believe that the extreme time demands and sleep deprivation compromise the delivery of quality medical care as well.

Exactly how the excess of demands on the intern affect the humanistic quality of the care delivered has received almost no empirical investigation. The chronic anger and cynicism suggested in Small's descriptive reports on the house officer's stress syndrome would suggest a decrease in the resident's ability and willingness to engage in a patient interaction characterized by concern and compassion. Indeed, the negative references to patients as "hits," "crocks," "turkeys," "gomers" is indicative of the resentment associated with having to interact with complex patients without immediately diagnosable and treatable medical illnesses in the face of having too many patients to care for in the first place. Given extreme time pressures, it is understandable why residents may prefer patients with clear-cut illnesses and injuries requiring straightforward treatment regimens. Such cases of clear-cut illness or trauma may also provide a greater sense of accomplishment to the physician preoccupied with crossing off a name on a long list of patients.

In the one empirical study of relevance to the effect of internship training on the humanitarianism of the intern, Adler et al. (1980) examined four classes of pediatric interns and found a less positive attitude toward patients after the internship year had been completed. In particular, satisfaction from helping patients and providing patient care became less rewarding. Additionally, at the end of the year interns considered social factors as less important determinants of health or illness, and for two of three intern classes, emotional components of the doctor-patient relationship were considered less important in patient care.

In sum, available knowledge suggests that both the medical student and the house officer, particularly the intern, are subjected to considerable stress. The training years seem to (1) impact negatively the medical trainee's own health habits such as proper sleep and eating habits, (2) decrease substantially the time available for meeting personal and social needs, and (3) show an association with an elevated risk for psychiatric symptomatology, particularly depression. There is a paucity of empirical data regarding how these stresses in the training years actually impact the quality of patient care delivered, particularly with regard to humanistic aspects of care delivery. The large body of literature on impairment in physicians in practice not reviewed here also raises questions about the potentially negative impact of the profession on the practitioner. The physician impairment literature focuses on depression and drug and alcohol abuse but unfortunately does little to address other aspects of impairment, such as the physician's inability to be genuinely concerned about the patient.

In addition to understanding how aspects of medical education and training may impede the development of humane, patient-oriented physicians, it is also important to remember that medical schools do not operate in isolation from the larger society. Indeed a number of forces negatively impinge on efforts to practice humane medicine, affecting not only medical schools but also the entire medical care delivery system. First, there has been a recognition that the rapid technological advances of medical science have created a critical shift in the doctor/patient relationship (Reiser 1982). Second, there has been a recognition that issues of cost effectiveness and cost containment are clearly impinging on the doctor/patient relationship.

This set of forces has been referred to by Bulger (1987) as the "bureaucratic theme." The concern here is that the profit motives of private industry may intervene in the traditional doctor/patient alliance where the physician is compelled solely by his or her concern for the welfare of the patient. In the bureaucratic delivery of health care services, the physician may find himself or herself responding not only to the welfare of the patient but also to the needs of the employing health care bureaucracy and corporation. Such a situation has the potential of driving a wedge into the traditional doctor/patient alliance. These same two themes were identified by Odegaard (1986), who wrote, "I do not want to see an ethical, beneficial, truly professional quality to the role they [physicians] play in caring for patients eroded by technological manipulation from within and bureaucratic management from without." Odegaard describes how the drive toward specialization and subspecialization has fragmented medical care, leaving the patient wondering who his or her physician is. The narrow perspective engendered by such specialization exposes the physician to the risk of being inadequate in dealing with the patient as a complex human being in a social context. It has also been observed that the rapid technological advances in medicine are creating ethical dilemmas of substantial proportions and that physicians are ill prepared to come to grips with many of these difficult dilemmas.

In the face of such threats to the doctor/patient alliance, it is important to understand how the medical profession has attempted to respond to these disquieting forces. One of the responses made by the medical profession has been to seriously reassess the medical model. It has begun to question the adequacy of this model, which emphasizes disease that is fully accounted for by deviations from normal biological variables, tends to view disease in terms of specific etiologies, and focuses on medicine as a biological science characterized by objectivity and neutrality. Indeed, by the 1970s and 1980s, many medical educators were calling for a broader view of the practice of medicine, one which attempted to understand the ill person in the context of everyday life and function. Engel (1977) argued for a more expansive model of human health and illness, one which expanded from a strictly biomedical model to a "biopsychosocial model" of human illness. Mishler et al. (1981) strongly argued for expanding the biomedical model to a broader model for medicine, one which incorporated social factors in understanding medical phenomena. Eisenberg and Kleinman (1981), who presented the case for the relevance of social science to medical practice, wrote: "The factors that determine who is and who is not a patient can only be understood by taking non-biological factors into account; patienthood is a social state, rather than simply a biological one." Psychosocial variables influence not only the social and personal meanings of illness but also the risk of becoming ill, the nature of the response to the illness, and its prognosis. Most recently, Tarlov (1988) constructed a strong case for a revised conceptual framework for medicine. In many circles, therefore, there was a growing consensus that a biological model of health and illness needed to be expanded to incorporate psychosocial influences on health and illness.

The need for physicians to be educated in the social sciences and humanities was also underscored by a report of the Panel on the General Professional Education of the Physician and College Preparation for Medicine. This panel, appointed in 1981 by the Association of American Medical Colleges, was asked to develop recommendations and strategies to improve the promotion of learning and the personal development of each medical student. It was also asked to stimulate broad discussions among medical school and college faculties about the philosophies and approaches to medical education. The report produced by this panel, commonly known as the GPEP Report, noted that given the continued prospect of an ever-increasing knowledge base for medicine and a very rapidly changing environment of health care delivery, there was a need for educating physicians who could solve problems, exhibit a capacity for continual learning, and relate to a complex social environment in which to practice medicine. The panel also observed that since environmental and lifestyle factors are becoming increasingly targeted as important determinants of health and illness, medical schools must place greater emphasis on teaching students to promote health and prevent disease. The thrust of many of the recommendations in the GPEP report, therefore, was to acknowledge the need for a broad perspective on medical practice. The need for broadly educated physicians was also underscored by Odegaard (1986), who convincingly advocated the need for increased education of physicians in the social sciences and humanities.

In recent years, the medical profession has also reiterated its commitment to practicing medicine with compassion and with a dedication to patients' well-being. The GPEP Report (Association of American Medical Colleges 1984), for example, in its introduction affirmed the belief that "every physician should be caring, compassionate and dedicated to patients—to keeping them well and to helping them when they are ill." The report further stated that "ethical sensitivity and moral integrity, combined with equanimity, humility, and self-knowledge are quintessential qualities of all physicians." Another major step forward in the reiteration of the tradition of a humanely based medical practice occurred when the American Board of Internal Medicine accepted a position paper of its Subcommittee on the Evaluation of Humanistic Qualities in the Internist (1983). In this position paper, the American Board of Internal Medicine in essence proposed that the public has a right to expect humanistic behavior in its physicians, and it further defined this as practicing medicine with integrity, respect, and compassion. The Board also advocated the development of methods to assess humanistic qualities in professional behavior during residency training. In the face of a deteriorating doctor/patient relationship, therefore, the medical profession itself saw the need to develop a model of medical practice that could more fully address the human context of health and illness and the need to strongly reaffirm its commitment to a compassionate and humane foundation of medical care.

These positive changes were also accompanied by other developments. There was an increasing willingness among medical schools to introduce topics of medical ethics into the curriculum (Association of American Medical Colleges 1986), and the medical education establishment also began to experiment with the development of innovative programs (Holzman 1986; Bates 1986). These innovations in medical education were probably motivated less by a concern about deficiencies in the humanistic attributes of medical trainees than they were from a concern about the increasingly unacceptable traditional methods of memorizing vast amounts of medical knowledge (Bok 1986). Nevertheless, these major changes in the educational programs of medical schools may well affect the humanistic aspects of the students' own experience and the development of humanistic attributes in the students' approaches to patient care. The final section of this book is devoted to a fuller description and examination of these innovative programs.

Most of the new educational programs, including those at the University of New Mexico and McMaster University in Canada and the new Pathway Program at Harvard, feature a small-group, problem-based learning format. Such innovative programs may turn out to be better suited to the human needs of the students, since there is considerably less likelihood of being lost in a crowded sea of faces and considerably more time is available for interaction with a faculty mentor, thus presumably rendering it easier to individualize instruction. By introducing patients onto the educational scene much earlier than the traditional programs and by making the material learned a natural spin-off of solving a patient's problem, much of the traditional frustration of the preclinical years may be avoided. In the newer programs, the relevance of basic science material is heightened and the students do not lose sight of the fact that medicine is about caring for patients, not just becoming experts in the biological sciences. In fact, there is some limited empirical evidence (Moore-West et al. 1986) that medical students in an innovative small-group, problem-based program found the learning environment to be more meaningful and more flexible and to be characterized by a more favorable emotional climate compared with students from a traditional program at the same school. Students in the innovative curriculum also did not show as much emotional distress as did students in the traditional curriculum. They also did not show as much of a decline in their ratings of closeness among students. These results suggest that innovative programs do have the potential for improving the human elements of the medical school experience of the students themselves; further evaluation, however, is needed to establish whether or not such educational programs affect the ways in which students subsequently treat patients.

It may also be significant that while showing an improved learning environment, these innovative programs do not seem to compromise the competence of the students. A recent review by Schmidt et al. (1987) of fifteen studies comparing educational outcomes of problem-based, community-oriented medical curricula with those of conventional programs showed little differences between them, although there may be a small advantage to conventional curricula on traditional measures of academic achievement and a small advantage to innovative curricula with respect to tasks related to clinical competence and the development of an inquisitive learning style. These programs also appear to influence students toward the selection of a primary care specialty.

Besides the development of innovative educational programs, several more limited attempts have been made to specifically teach humanistic patient care approaches within traditional medical schools. Gorlin and Zucker (1983), for example, reported on the development of a humanistic medicine program developed by the Department of Medicine at Mount Sinai School of Medicine. This program is based on the assumptions that all doctors, however humane, will at times have negative or positive feelings that can interfere with optimal professional judgment or action, and that freedom to acknowledge and discuss such feelings will help the doctor to maintain appropriately professional behavior. One aspect of the program is to use case discussions to focus on three elements: the patient's disease, the patient himself or herself, and the student's or resident's own response to the patient, the disease, and the health care system. There is also some use of co-teaching of residents by a seasoned internist and an experienced liaison psychiatrist. The acknowledgment of the doctor-in-training as a human being with feelings and reactions to the patients treated seems to facilitate the treatment of the patient as a human being with feelings. Wolf et al. (1987) developed an approach at the University of Michigan Medical School aimed at producing physicians who were compassionate as well as technically competent. To do this an effort was made to train medical students to address the emotional concerns that patients experience as a result of their medical problems. Students who received small-group instruction in addition to the large-group lectures offered were found to demonstrate the best ability to respond to the emotional concerns of patients. The small-group experiences were conducted with interviews of elderly nursing home residents, and students were introduced to listening and probing skills, to skills in empathic responding, and to the need for decreasing judgmental responses. Results of studies such as these suggest that it is possible to affect the degree of humaneness of the medical care delivered if careful instruction and modeling are directed toward this end.

While recent efforts at addressing concerns about the deterioration of the human qualities of medical care delivery are thus developing, it is difficult to know whether these concerns are infusing the medical education system or whether they are more appropriately characterized as existing in isolated pockets of influence. It would be reassuring to believe that interest in preserving and fostering humane qualities in the doctor/patient relationship is gaining widespread attention. Given the likelihood of continued technological progress, an increasing bureaucratization of health care delivery, and increasing concerns over health care financing, however, improvement in the doctor/patient relationship will face an uphill battle. Nevertheless, the protection of this important relationship is essential to satisfactory health care. It has also been suggested that the lack of humanistic behavior in physicians stems at least in part from their own experience in a less than optimally humane medical educational system. The factors identified as contributing to this less than optimal learning environment can be summarized as follows: (1) large classes with little opportunity for interaction with faculty, (2) exposure to massive amounts of information that may surpass the human ability to memorize it, (3) excessive time demands that result in the ignoring of student and resident needs for social interaction and recreation, (4) the presentation of large amounts of scientific material divorced from its relevance to patient care, (5) the lack of opportunity for significant interaction with patients during the early medical school years, (6) limited time for interaction with clinical faculty who are themselves preoccupied by pressures to obtain grant funds and publish as well as by pressures to generate substantial clinical income, (7) the experience of being subjected to excessively critical or humiliating evaluations of performance, and (8) the lack of opportunity for experiences in providing continuity of care to patients.

To educate and develop physicians capable of and motivated to practice medicine in a compassionate manner with the requisite abilities to understand psychosocial influences on illness and illness behavior, the following suggestions are offered:

1. Medical students must themselves be treated in a humane fashion, i.e., their educators must take into account human limitations with respect to learning capacities and must recognize that students and residents have human needs for social interaction and for recreation. Medical educators must also understand that students and residents need to be treated in a dignified manner, and educators must demonstrate some flexibility in responding to the individual needs of the physician in training.

2. Attention must be given during the training years to learning to be sensitive and responsive to human feelings, and this includes paying attention to the doctor's feelings and reactions as well as to those of patients. Students should have the opportunity to acknowledge their own feelings and reactions to patients and to learn how to ensure that these human feelings and reactions do not detract from their ability to provide professional care.

3. Adequate time for teaching and for quality patient interaction must be preserved; opportunities for exposure to seasoned, sensitive clinicians must be protected without allowing financial considerations to take precedence over all other considerations. The medical education system must

genuinely value the teaching activities of the faculty and must convey this valuing in promotion and tenure deliberations.

4. Students must be exposed to models of humanistic care. Students should have the opportunity to care for patients over extended time periods, and they should have the opportunity to attend to and understand patients' feelings about their illnesses, disabilities, and injuries.

5. New health care reimbursement mechanisms need to be experimented with in an effort to demonstrate the valuing not only of high tech procedures but also of the physicians' time spent in healing interpersonal interactions and in educating patients about health promoting behaviors.

In sum, if physicians-in-training are to acquire humane approaches to patient care they must be exposed to adequate models of caring behavior both in terms of the faculty caring for the students and in terms of the faculty caring for the patients. As Albert Schweitzer said, "Example is not the main thing in influencing others. It is the only thing."

REFERENCES

Adler, R., Werner, E. R., and Korsch, B. (1980). Systematic study of four years of internship. *Pediatrics,* 66, 1000–1008.
Alagna, S. W., and Morokoff, P. J. (1986). Beginning medical school: Determinants of male and female emotional reactions. *Journal of Applied Social Psychology,* 16, 348–360.
American Board of Internal Medicine, Subcommittee on Evaluation of Humanistic Qualities in the Internist (1983). Evaluation of humanistic qualities in the internist. *Annals of Internal Medicine,* 99, 720–724.
Association of American Medical Colleges (1984). Report of the Panel on the General Professional Education of the Physician and College Preparation for Medicine. Washington, D.C.: Association of American Medical Colleges.
Association of American Medical Colleges (1986). *Integrating Human Values Teaching Programs into Medical Students' Clinical Education.* Washington, D.C.: Association of American Medical Colleges.
Baca, E., Mennin, S. P., Kaufman, A., and Moore-West, M. (In press). A comparison between a problem-based, community-oriented track and traditional track within one medical school. In *Innovations in Medical Education: An Evaluation of Its Present Status* (ed. by T. Khattab, H. G. Schmidt, Z. Noonan, and E. Ezzat). New York: Springer.
Bates, P. (1986). The New Pathway at Harvard. *New Physician,* 35, 29–31.
Becker, H. S., and Geer, B. (1958). The fate of idealism in medical school. *American Sociological Review,* 23, 50–56.
Beckman, H. B., and Frankel, R. M. (1984). The effect of physician behavior on the collection of data. *Annals of Internal Medicine,* 101, 692–696.
Beeson, P. B. (1987). Making medicine a more attractive profession. *Journal of Medical Education,* 62, 116–125.
Bjorksten, O., Sutherland, S., Miller, C., and Stewart, T. (1983). *Journal of Medical Education,* 58, 759–767.
Bojar, S. (1961). Psychiatric problems of medical students. In *Emotional Problems of*

the Student (ed. by G. B. Blaine, Jr., and C. C. McArthur). New York: Appleton-Century-Crofts.

Bok, D. (1986) Professional schools. In *Higher Learning*. Cambridge, Mass.: Harvard University Press.

Boyle, B. P., and Coombs, R. H. (1971). Personality profiles related to emotional stress in the initial year of medical training. *Journal of Medical Education*, 46, 882–888.

Bulger, R. J. (1987). *Technology, Bureaucracy and Healing in America*. Iowa City: University of Iowa Press.

Clark, D. C., Salazar-Gruso, E., Grabler, P., and Fawcett, J. (1984). Predictors of depression during the first 6 months of internship. *American Journal of Psychiatry*, 141, 1095–1098.

Clark, E. J., and Rieker, P. P. (1986). Gender differences in relationships and stress of medical and law students. *Journal of Medical Education*, 61, 32–40.

Coburn, D., and Jovaises, A. V. (1975). Perceived sources of stress among first-year medical students. *Journal of Medical Education*, 50, 585–595.

Davies, B., Mowbray, R. M., and Jensen, D. (1968). A questionnaire survey of psychiatric symptoms in Australian medical students. *Australian and New Zealand Journal of Psychiatry*, 2, 46–53.

Duffy, D. L., Hamerman, D., and Cohen, M. A. (1980). Communication skills of house officers. *Annals of Internal Medicine*, 93, 354–357.

Edwards, M. T., and Zimet, C. N. (1976). Problems and concerns among medical students—1975. *Journal of Medical Education*, 51, 619–625.

Eisenberg, L. and Kleinman, A. (1981). *The Relevance of Social Sciences for Medicine*, vol. 1. Boston: D. Reidel.

Elliot, D. L., Girard, D. E., and Warren, L. (1985). Effect of gender on the emotional impact of internship (abstract). *Clinical Research*, 33, 43A.

Engel, G. (1977). The need for a new medical model: A challenge for biomedicine. *Science*, 196, 129–136.

Eron, L. D. (1955). The effect of medical education on medical students' attitudes. *Journal of Medical Education*, 30, 559–565.

Ford, C. V. (1983). Emotional distress in internship and residency: A questionnaire study. *Psychiatric Medicine*, 1, 143–150.

Ford, C. V., and Wentz, D. K. (1984). The internship year: A study of sleep, mood states, and psychophysiologic parameters. *Southern Medical Journal*, 77, 1435–1442.

Friedman, R. C., Kornfeld, D. S., and Bigger, T. J. (1973). Psychological problems associated with sleep deprivation in interns. *Journal of Medical Education*, 48, 436–441.

Firth-Cozens, J. (1987). Emotional distress in junior house officers. *British Medical Journal*, 295, 533–536.

Girard, D. E., Elliott, D. L., Hickman, P. H., Sparr, L., Clarke, N. G., Warren, L., and Koski, J. (1986). The internship—A prospective investigation of emotions and attitudes. *Western Journal of Medicine*, 144, 93–98.

Glickman, R. M. (1988). House-staff training—The need for careful reform. *New England Journal of Medicine*, 318, 780–782.

Gorlin, R., and Zucker, H. D. (1983). Physicians' reactions to patients: A key to teaching humanistic medicine. *New England Journal of Medicine*, 308, 1059–1063.

Green, S. A., and Miyai, K. (1986). The impact of medical school on the student with respect to interpersonal relationships and lifestyles. *Journal of Medical Education*, 61, 177–178.

Greer, D. S. (1987). Review of *Dear Doctor: A Personal Letter to a Physician. Journal of Medical Education*, 62, 611–613.

Holzman, D. (1986). Med schools test problem-solving. *Insight,* 9, 60–62.
Hsu, K. and Marshall, V. (1987). Prevalence of depression and distress in a large sample of Canadian residents, interns and fellows. *American Journal of Psychiatry,* 144, 1561–1566.
Huebner, L. A., Royer, J. A., and Moore, J. (1981). The assessment and remediation of dysfunctional stress in medical school. *Journal of Medical Education,* 56, 547–558.
Hunter, R. C. A., Prince, R. H., and Schwartzman, A. E. (1961). Comments on emotional disturbances in a medical undergraduate population. *Journal of the American Medical Association,* 83, 989–992.
Kay, J., Howard, T., and Welch, G. (1980). Health habits of medical students: Some perils of the profession. *Journal of the American College Health Association,* 28, 238–39.
Kellner, R., Wiggins, R. J. and Pathak, D. (1986). Distress in medical and law students. *Comprehensive Psychiatry,* 27, 220–223.
Kelly, J. A., St. Lawrence, J. S., Smith, S., Jr., Hood, H. V., and Cook, D. J. (1987). Medical students' attitudes towards AIDS and homosexual patients. *Journal of Medical Education,* 62, 549–556.
Krupat, E. (1986). A delicate imbalance: Has modern medicine, with all its technological advances, lost sight of the human element in healing? *Psychology Today,* 20, 22–26.
Landau, C., Hall, S., Wartman, S. A., and Macko, M. B. (1986). Stress in social and family relationships during the medical residency. *Journal of Medical Education,* 61, 654–660.
Lloyd, C., and Gartrell, N. K. (1981). Sex differences in medical student mental health. *American Journal of Psychiatry,* 138, 1346–1351.
Lloyd, C., and Gartrell, N. K. (1983). A further assessment of medical school stress. *Journal of Medical Education,* 58, 964–967.
Lloyd, C., and Gartrell, N. K. (1984). Psychiatric symptoms in medical students. *Comprehensive Psychiatry,* 552–565.
McCue, J. D. (1985). The distress of internship: Causes and prevention. *New England Journal of Medicine,* 312, 449–452.
Mellinkoff, S. M. (1987). Introduction to the art: Perceptions in New Zealand, Australia, and the United Kingdom. *Pharos,* 50, 8–10.
Mishler, E. G., Amarasingham, L. R., Hauser, S. T., Liem, R., Osherson, S. D., and Waxler, N. E. (1981). *Social Contexts of Health, Illness, and Patient Care.* Cambridge: Cambridge University Press.
Moore-West, M., Harrington, D. L., Mennin, S. P., and Kaufman, A. (1986). Distress and attitudes toward the learning environment: Effects of a curriculum innovation. *Proceedings of the Annual Conference on Research in Medical Education,* 25, 293–300.
Moore-West, M., Jackson, R., Kaufman, A., Obenshein, S. S., Galey, W., Donnell, M., and West, D. (1986). Reduced stress in medical education: An outcome of altered learning environment. Paper presented at the annual meeting of the American Psychiatric Association, Washington, D.C.
Muller, S. (1984). *Introduction to Physicians for the Twenty-first Century: Report of the Panel on the General Professional Education of the Physician and College Preparation for Medicine.* Washington, D.C.: Association of American Medical Colleges.
Odegaard, C. E. (1986). *Dear Doctor: A Personal Letter to a Physician.* Menlo Park, Calif.: Henry J. Kaiser Family Foundation.
Osler, W. (1921). The Evaluation of Modern Medicine. A series of lectures delivered at Yale University on the Silliman Foundation in April, 1913, p. 58.
Pepitone-Areola-Rockwell, F., Rockwell, D., and Core, N. (1981). Fifty-two medical student suicides. *American Journal of Psychiatry,* 138, 198–201.

Petersdorf, R. G. (1986). Medical education for the future: A mandate for change. *Internist*, 27, 17–20.

Petersdorf, R. G. (1988). Balancing concerns for quality patient care and quality residency training. *Journal of Medical Education*, 63, 410–411.

Pitts, F. N., Winokur, G., and Stewart, M. A. (1961). Psychiatric syndromes, anxiety symptoms and responses to stress in medical students. *American Journal of Psychiatry*, 118, 333–340.

Platt, F. W., and McMath, S. C. (1979). Clinical hypocompetence: The interview. *Annals of Internal Medicine*, 91, 898–902.

Reiser, S. J. (1982). Technology and the eclipse of individualism in medicine. *Pharos*, 45, 10–15.

Reuben, D. B. (1985). Depressive symptoms in medical house officers: Effects of level of training and work rotation. *Archives of Internal Medicine*, 145, 286–288.

Rosenberg, P. P. (1971). Students' perceptions and concerns during their first year in medical school. *Journal of Medical Education*, 46, 211–218.

Roeske, N. C. A. (1981). Stress and the physician. *Psychiatric Annals*, 11, 245–258.

Rosenberg, D. A., and Silver, H. K. (1984) Medical student abuses: An unnecessary and preventable cause of stress. *Journal of the American Medical Association*, 251, 739–742.

Saslow, G. (1956). Psychiatric problems of medical students. *Journal of Medical Education*, 31, 27–33.

Schmidt, H. G., Dauphinee, W. D., and Patel, V. L. (1987). Comparing the effects of problem-based and conventional curricula in an international sample. *Journal of Medical Education*, 62, 305–315.

Schwartz, M. A., and Wiggins, D. (1985). Science, humanism, and the nature of medical practice: A phenomenological view. *Perspectives in Biology and Medicine*, 28, 331–361.

Shanfield, S. B., and Benjamin, G. A. H. (1984). Psychiatric distress in medical students: A macroscopic analysis. Paper presented at the annual meeting of the American Psychiatric Association, Los Angeles.

Small, G. W. (1981). House officer stress syndrome. *Psychosomatics*, 22, 860–869.

Tarlov, A. R. (1988). The rising supply of physicians and the pursuit of better health. *Journal of Medical Education*, 63, 94–107.

Uliana, R. L., Hubbell, F. A., Wyle, F. A., and Gordon, G. H. (1984). Mood changes during the internship. *Journal of Medical Education*, 59, 118–123.

Vaillant, G. E., Sobowole, N. C., and MacArthur, C. (1972). Some psychological vulnerabilities of physicians. *New England Journal of Medicine*, 287, 372–375.

Valko, R., and Clayton, P. (1975). Depression in the internship. *Diseases of the Nervous System*, 36, 26–29.

Vitaliano, D. P., Russo, J., Carr, J. E., and Heerwagen, J. H. (1984). Medical school pressures and their relationship to anxiety. *Journal of Nervous and Mental Disease*, 172, 730–736.

Whalen, J. P. (1987). Participation of medical students in the care of patients with AIDS. *Journal of Medical Education*, 62, 53–54.

Wolf, F. M., Woolliscroft, J. O., Calhoun, J. G., and Boxer, G. J. (1987). A controlled experiment in teaching students to respond to patients' emotional concerns. *Journal of Medical Education*, 62, 25–34.

Wolf, T. M., and Kisling, G. E. (1984). Changes in lifestyle characteristics, health and mood of freshman medical students. *Journal of Medical Education*, 59, 806–815.

Zocolillo, M., Murphy, G. E., and Wetzel, R. D. (1986). Depression among medical students. *Journal of Affective Disorder*, 11, 91–96.

Part Three

Toward a More Humane Medicine

LESSONS FROM THE PAST AND RECENT INNOVATIONS IN MEDICAL EDUCATION

In part three, an effort is made to place current attempts to sensitize prospective physicians to humanistic issues in an historical and societal context. In the first essay, Regina Morantz-Sanchez visits the nineteenth century to detail how women's medical colleges and early prominent women physicians addressed the human aspects of medical practice, documenting, in fact, the major role played by women in advocating the art as well as the science of medicine. Morantz-Sanchez reminds the reader of how these early women emphasized the role of sympathy, nurturance, and intuition in the care of patients. The second essay of the section, by Maggie Moore-West and her colleagues, provides a valuable overview and summary of recent innovations in medical education which, among other aims, have attempted to humanize medical practice. These recent innovations have generally taken one of two approaches. The first approach has re-emphasized community-oriented primary care in order to foster among practitioners a greater appreciation of both the psychosocial context in which the patient lives and the importance of preventive aspects of health care. The second approach has emphasized problem-based learning in order to provide the human context for the study of basic science. The essay also discusses how medical faculty have been prepared to participate in such innovative developments. Finally, the essay provides a preliminary assessment of the efficacy of such innovations.

The third and fourth essays describe programmatic efforts aimed at reducing stress among house staff and providing them with a more humane setting in which to work. The third focuses on pediatric residents and discusses how faculty must assist their residents in adapting to the stressors inherent in medical care delivery. The fourth describes an experimental intervention on a medical oncology unit aimed at reducing stress among house staff. One very interesting feature of this program was the demonstration that the improvement in the emotional reserves of the house staff had a positive impact upon the humane aspects of patient care.

EIGHT

Women's Contribution to Medical Education

A Nineteenth-Century Case Study

REGINA MORANTZ-SANCHEZ

Health care has become an industry that absorbs an ever-increasing proportion of the nation's wealth. Increases in medical costs outdistance
general inflation year after year. Many persons have begun to question the
benefits of increasingly refined technological approaches to the basic problems of health. In the final analysis, relatively little progress has been made
in treating the twin killers of modern life, cancer and heart disease. In
addition, we face a new plague of epidemic proportions—AIDS—which
thus far has responded hardly at all to the efforts of laboratory scientists to
bring it under control. Sickness still disproportionately affects the poor.

In spite of these troubling realities, the ideology of science retains
enormous cultural power and resonance. This ideology puts enormous
faith in the collection of "objective" data, fosters laboratory experiments
under suitable controls, urges the precise measuring and counting of
results, the repetition of protocols, and the publication of findings. It tends
to devalue all forms of knowledge that cannot be subsumed under the
category of "hard facts." Although most careful estimates indicate that the
medical system (doctors, drugs, and hospitals) affects only about 10 percent
of the nation's health measured by the standard indices of infant mortality,
adult morbidity, and longevity, it is the medical system that gets the most
scrutiny from policy makers. The social, environmental, and occupational
causes of illness—which account for the largest proportion of morbidity
and mortality but cannot be measured or reproduced in the laboratory—
receive comparatively scant attention (Wildavsky 1977, p. 105). Medical
education has for at least half a century reflected this myopic approach to
the training of practitioners.

As a result, critics from within the profession have in the last decade

117

joined forces with the lay public and detractors from a variety of disciplines to decry a "model of disease no longer adequate" to its scientific tasks or social responsibilities. "Medicine's crisis," the psychiatrist George L. Engel has written, "stems from the logical inference that since 'disease' is defined in terms of somatic parameters, physicians need not be concerned with psychosocial issues which lie outside medicine's responsibility and authority." Engel (1977) deplores the persistence of a "mind-body dualism" in medical thinking which assumes that the whole can be understood "both materially and conceptually by reconstituting the parts." He warns that the present approach to disease "neglects the patient" and that younger physicians increasingly are forced to confront the contradictions between the "excellence of their biomedical background" and the "weakness of their qualifications . . . essential for good patient care."

To the historian of women physicians, much of this criticism has a familiar ring. This is so because a little less than a century ago, women physicians struggled with changes in medicine which threatened to revolutionize its organization and practice and called into question their rationale for entry into the profession. Perhaps a closer look at how they faced this crisis can offer some insight into contemporary difficulties. We will see that women physicians tended to represent a certain approach to the teaching and practice of medicine, one which was rapidly being devalued in the heady and expectant intellectual atmosphere of the late nineteenth-century bacteriological revolution.

In the middle of the nineteenth century, the medical profession was immature, lacking most of the identifying characteristics that would be taken for granted seventy years later. It shared no common intellectual base and was plagued by competing sects with contending theories on the causes and treatment of disease. Educational standards were haphazard except in one respect: they were uniformly low. Generally unable to control entry into the field, physicians were forced to stand by as women and other "undesirables" were licensed to practice. Weak and ineffectual professional societies had yet to develop either a strict professional ethos or a set of shared ethical assumptions.

Even more significant, the physician's approach to treatment was shaped by a traditional system of belief and behavior shared by doctor and patient alike. Central to this system was a holistic view of the body which defined sickness as the maladaptive state of the entire organism: the body out of step with its environment. Individual body parts were believed to be integrally connected: thus emotional stress could cause indigestion just as surely as indigestion could bring on emotional distress. The dictates of such a system demanded that the physician know his or her patient well. The "art" of medicine lay with the doctor's ability to select the proper drug in the proper dose to bring on the proper physiological effect. Self-respecting practitioners knew that they must be familiar not only with the patient's history and unique physical identity but with the family's constitutional idiosyncrasies as well. These were assessed along with relevant environmental, climatic, and developmental conditions.

It should come as no surprise that under such a system the locus of practice and treatment was the patient's own home. Indeed, doctors most often treated entire families, and in emphasizing the sacredness of personal ties between doctors and patients, early medical ethics merely echoed on another plane a medical theory that stressed the relevance of family history to clinical judgments.

Though this therapeutic framework was labeled scientific, no physician in the nineteenth century would have minimized the importance of intuitive factors in successful diagnosis and treatment. Hence the words *medical science* harbored a somewhat different meaning than they do today. "The model of the body, and of health and disease," Charles Rosenberg (1981, pp. 10–11) has observed, "was all-inclusive, antireductionist, capable of incorporating every aspect of man's life in explaining his physical condition. Just as man's body interacted continuously with his environment, so did his mind with his body, his morals with his health. The realm of causation in medicine was not distinguishable from the realm of meaning in society generally." As Professor Henry Hartshorne (1872, pp. 6–7) put it to the graduating class of the Woman's Medical College of Pennsylvania in 1872, "It is not always the most logical, but often the most discerning physician who succeeds best at the bedside. Medicine is indeed a science, but its practice is an art. Those who bring the quick eye, the receptive ear, and delicate touch, intensified, all of them, by a warm sympathetic temperament . . . may use the learning of laborious accumulators, often, better than they themselves could do."

Ironically, when advances in the laboratory began to discredit traditional heavy dosing, emphasizing instead the self-limiting nature of most diseases, the "art" of medical practice temporarily became even more important. Often skeptical of his or her own ability to intervene, many a physician sought merely to minimize pain and anxiety and "wait on nature." Such a situation made some members of the profession particularly receptive to the entrance of women.

For their part, women entered the field by championing an extremely powerful paradigm of ideal womanhood which became so embedded in nineteenth-century American culture that one easily finds traces of it today. Though women physicians did not singlehandedly invent the ideal, they believed in it, helped to define it, and used it to achieve their own ends. Its features have been painstakingly explored by historians over the past decade (see Walsh 1977 and Morantz-Sanchez 1985). According to its dictates, the central organizing metaphor for women's lives—their mission in society, so to speak—was motherhood. Though the Victorian sanctification of motherhood could sequester women in the family at home, it just as often served as a persuasive justification for a more integral role for women in society at large. Indeed, women did not always have to become mothers in

the physiological sense. Thus Elizabeth Blackwell, a leader in the movement to train women in medicine and a person with strong ideas about
medical education, could speak repeatedly of "the spiritual power of a
maternity" which all true physicians—male or female—must possess (Blackwell 1889, pp. 10, 13, and 21). By this term she meant something very akin
to Erik Erikson's idea of generativity, a concept which he defined as "the
concern in establishing and guiding the next generation" (Erikson 1950).
Like Erikson, Blackwell interpreted the spiritual power of maternity in the
broadest possible terms. Not only physicians, but all mankind must learn
the lessons it had to teach, whether individuals actually had children or not.

Well into the twentieth century, women physicians were reiterating this
theme. "Being women as well as physicians," acknowledged Margaret
Vaupel Clark, president of the Iowa State Society of Medical Women, "we
share with our sex in the actual and potential motherhood of the race.
Being women we make common cause with all women. . . . And being
women and mothers, our first and closest and dearest interest is the child"
(Clark 1915, p. 128).

Wedding this cultural paradigm to traditional assumptions about the
role of the physician, female medical leaders and their supporters fash-
ioned a formidable argument for training women in medicine. If the
doctor's responsibilities were integrally linked to the family, who better
than scientifically trained women could monitor family health? "Ladies,"
the dean of the Woman's Medical College of Pennsylvania told a graduating
class in 1858, "it is for the very purpose of making home enjoyments more
complete that you have been delegated today to bear health and hope to the
abodes you enter" (Preston 1858, p. 10). "Our medical profession," Elizabeth Blackwell observed, "has not yet fully realized the special and weighty
responsibility which rests upon it to watch over the cradle of the race; to see
to it that human beings are well born, well nourished, and well educated."
Such work, she believed, was "especially encumbent upon women physicians," who better understood "the all important character of parentage in
its influence upon . . . the race" (Blackwell 1896, p. 253).

Moreover, given the demands made on a good practitioner, women had
a natural vocation for it. They were, argued Dr. Marie Zakrzewska, "by
nature sympathetic and more caretaking in sickness" (Vietor 1924, p. 376).
"The True physician," wrote Angenette Hunt in her graduating thesis from
the Woman's Medical College of Pennsylvania, needed "gentleness, patience, quick perceptions, natural instinct which is often surer than science,
deep sympathy." All these qualities, Hunt believed, "belong to the sex in an
eminent degree" (Hunt 1851).

With the bacteriological revolution at the end of the nineteenth century,
doctors increasingly confronted a tension between "art" and science in
medicine, a tension which women doctors felt most acutely. They had
entered the profession believing in women's special abilities to alleviate pain
and suffering. They had wrestled with their dual identities as women and

as doctors. They had emphasized the importance of prevention over cure and the duty of doctors to bring about social reform. Yet, until bacteriology injected a specific kind of science into medical practice, one characterized by an approach to knowledge which was allegedly dispassionate, precise, and subject to suitable tests of proof, evidence, and the collective criticisms of the scientific community, they functioned in an atmosphere colored by an older concept of professionalism, one accepted by both sexes, which maintained a place for subjective forms of knowing and stressed the therapeutic powers of moral and social concerns. To someone like Elizabeth Blackwell, bacteriology threatened to destroy this world, undermining in the process women doctors' raison d'etre. Indeed, Blackwell's ideas on medical education and practice represent a particularly interesting historical strain in the thinking of women doctors, one which was, in spite of its shortcomings, remarkably prescient in its understanding of the direction medicine was moving.

Rankled by the exaggerated claims of the early microbe hunters, Blackwell devoted considerable attention in her later writings to the dangers of medical materialism and the question of what the pursuit of science really entailed. In her view, bacteriology could never fit her definition of "true science," because its theory of disease causation was overly simplistic. Bacteriologists consistently overlooked the connection between the mind and the body. "We can take a steam-engine or a watch to pieces, examine their parts, repair them, and put them together again," she wrote in a vein remarkably reminiscent of the words of George L. Engel with which I began this article. "But a living thing cannot be treated in the same way" (Blackwell 1898, p. 135). To regard human beings as simply "material bodies" without considering the effect of the mental state on the health of those bodies was bad science and consequently bad medicine. "Sanitary law," she argued, "teaches us that disease is produced by many causes, not solely by a specific microbe" (Blackwell 1891, pp. 50 and 75).

It followed that if disease was multicausational, the true scientist needed to pursue, not only objective but what we would now call subjective data. "Science is not . . . an accumulation of isolated facts, or of facts torn from their natural relations," Blackwell insisted. "For science unites and demands the exercise of our various faculties as well as of our senses. . . . Scientific method requires that all the factors which concern the subject of research shall be duly considered. . . ." Elsewhere in the same essay she elaborated on what some of those other factors might be: "The facts of affection, companionship, sympathy, justice . . . exercise a powerful influence over the physical organization of all living creatures" (1898, pp. 126–130).

Moreover, laboratory research too often entailed research without patients. For Blackwell, such an approach to medicine was almost a contradiction in terms. While experimental investigators viewed themselves as progressives whose discoveries would rapidly advance the treatment of disease, she sided with the more traditional of her colleagues who still venerated a personal, humane style of interaction oriented toward the individual patient. A new image of the medical scientist emerged at the end of the nineteenth century—an individual who was calculating, manipulative, and objectively detached from the object of study, and it troubled her to the end of her life. It seemed a wholesale rejection of the interpersonal dimension of medicine, on which her entire conception of the physician's task rested.

When she paused to consider the mission of medical education, Blackwell, herself the founder of two women's medical schools, proved to be a devoted supporter of medical research—in the form of clinical casework, postmortem and gross pathology, pathological chemistry, microscopic anatomy, and other types of patient-centered investigations. Such study, she believed, would prove essential in providing the raw data on which inductions regarding the causes and prevention of disease could be based. "In medicine," she told students at the London School of Medicine for Women in 1889, "anatomy, physiology and chemistry are the primary studies . . . on which the skill of the future physicians so largely depends" (1889, p. 15). "The conquest of pain and diminution of nervous shock in necessary surgical operations, the disappearance of blood-poisoning, hospital gangrene, and erysipelas . . . are . . . the direct outcome of persevering and skilful clinical observation, of careful work in the laboratory, of humane experiment . . ." (1898, p. 105).

Unfortunately bacteriologists had inspired innovations in medical education which persistently troubled her. Particularly disturbing was the introduction of vivisection, a teaching method which she considered not only dangerous but also "erroneous." Because of the necessity of knowingly inflicting pain on living, sentient beings, animal experimentation represented to Blackwell an attempt to seek good ends through immoral means. She felt such an approach could lead only to disastrous professional consequences. Vivisection would encourage the experimenter to detach himself or herself from the object of the research, she predicted, and it could only harden its practitioners. If taught extensively in medical schools, it would surely render students incapable of mustering "that intelligent sympathy with suffering, which is a fundamental quality in the good physician." The outcome would be an inability to identify with patients, especially the sick poor, who, she warned with extraordinary foresight, might soon be regarded as "clinical material." For Blackwell, "the attitude of the student and doctor to the sick poor" was the final test "of the true physician" (1891, p. 43; 1889, p. 13).

Blackwell was not an isolated thinker among late nineteenth century women physicians. Admittedly, only a handful of them opposed bacteriology with her force or conviction; indeed, most welcomed the new discoveries. Yet her critique of objective, value-free science continued to be shared by many of her female colleagues well into the era of experimental inquiry, technology, and specialization. One did not need to oppose vivisection to worry about the dehumanizing effects of medical education.

I would suggest that there were two distinguishing features of female medical education in the late nineteenth and early twentieth centuries. The first was an emphasis on prevention. The second was the attempt to teach students that the doctor-patient relationship was absolutely central to diagnosis and treatment, while technological interventions, though important, were to be used selectively and secondarily (Brody 1987). In other words, most women physicians remained wedded to a belief in the psychosocial components of illness, in spite of increasing pressures to discount such an approach.

The theme of preventive medicine recurs like a refrain in the writings of early generations of women doctors. Marie Zakrzewska, for example, founder of the New England Hospital for Women and Children, justified her use of placebos by her willingness to teach people "how to keep well." Others gave lectures on physiology and health to the public. The early women's medical schools and hospitals built such concerns into their curricula. The medical school of the New York Infirmary for Woman and Children boasted proudly of the first course in hygiene (preventive medicine) offered anywhere in the country. A year before the founding of the school, the hospital had established the office of "sanitary vistor," an individual designated by the hospital to give special attention to the physician's teaching role. The position was usually filled by a young medical graduate wishing to gain further clinical experience. The work entailed going into the homes of the poor, checking on ventilation, cleanliness, diet, and general hygiene, and giving families advice on how to keep themselves healthy (Morantz-Sanchez 1985, pp. 75 and 216).

Other women's insitutions followed suit. In Cleveland and Philadelphia, the Woman's Hospitals sent interns into patients' homes. Physicians, revealed the Cleveland Hospital's Annual Report of 1882, did not confine their work "entirely to curing the sick" but also offered "instruction . . . in the laws of health" and in the "care and diet of children." Similarly, the Mary Harris Thompson Hospital in Chicago had female physicians as medical visitors who did "many things for their improvement besides administering medicines for a present illness" when they went "into the homes of the poor" (Morantz-Sanchez 1985, p. 216).

The teaching and practice of obstetrics was another area that reflected women doctors' strong concern with both preventive medicine and the psychosocial perameters of disease. In the last third of the nineteenth century, this branch of medical education lagged pitifully behind other subjects. Most institutions remained content to teach midwifery solely through didactic lectures. In contrast, Dr. Anna Broomall organized an outpatient department connected to the Woman's Hospital of the Woman's Medical College of Pennsylvania in 1876. Eventually this facility offered the first prenatal care in the country. Each medical student was responsible for the independent management of at least six obstetric cases before she qualified for the degree. The Woman's Medical College of the New York Infirmary provided a similar experience in obstretrics and gynecology. The 1888 faculty minutes refer to a requirement demanding that every student attend at least twelve cases before graduation (Morantz-Sanchez 1985, pp. 78–79).

Moreover, my comparison of male and female therapeutics at two Boston obstetrical hospitals during this same period revealed that, although differences in the *mechanics* of obstetrical practice were minimal, subtle but meaningful variations in physician-patient interaction may have made the experience of being treated by a woman physician a more positive one for the patient. For example, women doctors made rounds more often than the men and prescribed mild, supportive therapies, while their male counterparts did not. The women concerned themselves with their patients' social situations. Many an unmarried mother was settled in a job after she left the hospital, and countless poor patients were kept long after their recovery until proper housing could be found for them.

An intern at the female-run hospital during the 1870s reported a "ceaseless round of care, work, and anxiety." "The Maternity is the saddest of places to me," she wrote a friend. "Most of the women are unmarried, and except for the respectability of the thing, by far the greater number had better not be—the Husbands being brutal wretches who abuse them in every way." Proud of the efforts of the hospital's lady managers to help such unfortunate women find work and a home, she concluded, "I have always been interested in such work . . . and I am very glad, as you may imagine, to take any part in it." Even today, studies reveal that women physicians often spend more time with their patients and usually take a more thorough history (Morantz-Sanchez 1985, pp. 225–231 and 212).

A fascinating piece of evidence which may be taken as perhaps illustrative of many women physicians' holistic sense of their task as obstetricians can be found in a remarkable little volume of short stories and nonfiction essays entiled *Daughters of Aesculapius,* published in 1897 by the medical students and alumnae of the Woman's Medical College of Pennsylvania. The book speaks eloquently of the deepest concerns young women physicians shared at a time when they contended with a profession gradually taking on its modern face. In the story "Mater Dolorosa—Mater Felix," Anna Fullerton, class of 1882, writes of a sensitive, unmarried hospital resident who draws out from a beautiful young obstetrical patient the confession that her three-day-old baby is illegitimate. Able to intuit the inner goodness in this desperate unfortunate, the doctor manages to convince the wealthy young seducer to marry his mistress. The tale ends several years later with a visit from the woman—now a happy, refined, and elegant matron—requesting that the doctor see her through her second pregnancy. When the young lady thanks the woman physician for altering her fate, the latter responds that it was Providence who chose to do good through the "humble instrumentality of a woman doctor."

Female medical educators continually stressed the importance in therapeutics of the art of medical practice, eschewing biological reductionism. Sarah Adamson Dolley urged her students to meet patients "as something more than a static entity or dynamic quantity whose muscles, nerves, and joints are not simply a bundle of levers, pulleys and hinges, but are the instruments of that mysterious something which we call life." Mary E. Bates was particularly disgusted by a seminar on gynecologic surgery sponsored by her state medical society. The speakers, she complained, "limited their attacks to the offending . . . uterus," while practically ignoring the patient. Similarly, Dean Clara Marshall emphasized this point to her graduating classes in Philadelphia. Study people as well as diseases, she warned. "A distinguished physician has said 'there are no diseases, only patients,' " she told a group of students in 1879, and you will often reach patients and cure them too, by a scientific use of your humanity." Susan Dimock, a brilliant young surgeon at the New England Hospital, frequently commented that if she were asked "to do without sympathy or medicine, I should say do without medicine." "A woman physician sees life without its mask," observed the surgeon Rosalie Slaughter Morton. "[She] gets closer to the inner thought of other women in understanding the many domestic and social factors in illness . . . because her mother heart has scientific facts to support intuition and sympathy" (Morantz-Sanchez 1985, pp. 209–211).

There is also evidence that the female faculty at the women's medical schools understood that the best way to produce humane practitioners was to create a humane and supportive atmosphere for their students. This important insight has all too often been lost in contemporary medical institutions determined to educate practitioners who presumably must be rational, aggressively objective, comfortably detached from the object of study (in this case the patient), and without personal lives of their own. In contrast, medical education at the all-female schools in the nineteenth century may well have been less authoritarian than at the men's institutions. Female faculty consciously served as role models, and the significance to younger women of such exposure should not be minimized. Testimony proliferates in letters and diaries of both the professionalism and underlying warmth of such teachers. Anna Wessel Williams, while she took note of the impressive medical record of Professor Chevalier, who taught chemistry at the New York Infirmary, also recalled that Chevalier took "a personal interest" in her, giving her hints as to how she should dress and do her hair. Despite Mary Putnam Jacobi's reputation as an energetically brilliant and demanding teacher, she too gave Williams support and advice and helped her through several crucial decisions. She often gently "exposed our ignorance," remembered Williams, but always "in such a way that we were not so much depressed as encouraged to make it less" (Morantz-Sanchez 1985, pp. 111–112).

Similar memories abound of the Woman's Medical College of Pennsylvania faculty. Ann Preston, concerned about broadening her students in all ways, often took them to lectures by Lucy Stone and Ralph Waldo Emerson. Emmeline Cleveland combined calm, dignity, warmth, and femininity with undeniable professional competence to create a figure of quiet charisma for those students who knew her. Cleveland's successor in the chair of obstetrics, Anna Broomall, a particularly busy professor and practitioner, was remembered by her students for her compassion and her loyalty to family relationships. "This loyalty," wrote a student, "was consistently applied when the families of her assistants needed them. Work never pressed so hard, that we could not go to our families if illness or trouble came to our homes" (Morantz-Sanchez 1985, p. 112).

The Victorian world in which early women physicians lived sharply delineated the rational from the intuitive, head from heart, and identified the one with men and the other with women. Therefore, it should come as no surprise to us that their ideas often reflected this gender dichotomy. Elizabeth Blackwell, for example, was unequivocal in connecting bacteriology to the "male intellect." Indeed, she warned her women students that "it is not blind imitation of men, nor thoughtless acceptance of whatever may be taught by them that is required, for this would endorse the widespread error that the race is men" (Blackwell 1889, pp. 9–10). It follows that she believed the task of preserving an alternative, more nurturing view of medicine would fall primarily to women. Yet, however close she came to special pleading on the grounds of female biology, she stubbornly maintained a theory of physician-patient relationships which was not gender bound. Like some contemporary feminists, she believed that it was the tasks assigned to women—particularly mothering—that produced their social vision. That vision was as essential to medicine as the medical profession was to society at large. What women had learned must be taught to everyone, but especially to physicians.

It is time for us to rescue the activity of caring from the stranglehold of the extreme gender differentiation that characterized medical and scientific culture in the late nineteenth and first half of the twentieth centuries. Caring is not "owned" by women any more than rationality is exclusively the province of men. To the degree that female medical educators' teachings in the nineteenth century fostered the belief in such differences, they did the medical profession no service. Yet their accomplishments—a holistic and humane approach to medical education and practice—surely can serve us now as an alternative historical tradition well worth the attention of their professional heirs, male and female alike.

REFERENCES

Blackwell, E. (1889). The influence of women in the profession of medicine. (1898). Scientific method in biology. (1891). Erroneous method of medical education. In E. Blackwell (ed.), *Essays in Medical Sociology;* 2. New York: Arno, 1972.

Blackwell, E. 1896. *Pioneer Work in Opening the Medical Profession to Women.* New York: Longman Green.

Brody, H. (1987). *Stories of Sickness.* New Haven, Conn.: Yale University Press.

Clark, M. V.(1915). Medical women's contribution to the education of mothers. *Woman's Medical Journal*, 25, 126–128.

Daughters of Aesculapius: Stories Written by Alumnae and Students of the Women's Medical College of Pennsylvania (1897). Philadelphia: Woman's Medical College of Pennsylvania.

Engel, G. (1977). The need for a new medical model: A challenge for biomedicine. *Science*, 196, 128–135.

Erikson, E. (1950). *Childhood and Society.* New York: Norton.

Hartshorne, H. (1872). Valedictory Address. Philadelphia: Woman's Medical College of Pennsylvania.

Hunt, A. (1851). *The True Physician.* Thesis, Woman's Medical College of Pennsylvania, Philadelphia.

Morantz-Sanchez, R. (1985). *Sympathy and Science: Women Physicians in American Medicine.* New York: Oxford University Press.

Preston, A. (1858). Valedictory Address. Philadelphia: Woman's Medical College of Pennsylvania.

Rosenberg, C. (1981). The therapeutic revolution: Medicine, meaning and social change in nineteenth-century America. In C. Rosenberg and M. Vogel (eds.), *The Therapeutic Revolution: Essays on the Social History of American Medicine.* Philadelphia: University of Pennsylvania Press.

Vietor, A. (ed.) (1924). *A Woman's Quest: The Life of Marie E. Zakrzewska, M.D.* New York: D. Appleton.

Walsh, M. (1977). *Doctors Wanted: No Women Need Apply: Sexual Barriers in the Medical Profession, 1835–1977.* New Haven, Conn.: Yale University Press.

Wildavsky, A. (1977). "Doing Better and Feeling Worse: The Political Pathology of Health Policy." In J. H. Knowles (ed.), *Doing Better and Feeling Worse: Health in the United States.* New York: Norton.

NINE

Innovations in Medical Education

Enhancing Humanism through the
Educational Process

MAGGIE MOORE-WEST, MARTHA REGAN-SMITH,
ALLEN DIETRICH, AND DONALD O. KOLLISCH

> I don't actually have the hard statistics, but
> everybody says, it's a general understanding,
> that we're doing much better than last year
> did. If anybody thinks that it is for any reason
> except that there were quizzes every week,
> they're sorely, sadly mistaken. I really think
> that it was punitive. People rise to the level
> they are expected to rise to. And here every
> week you were expected to learn and you
> couldn't put it away. We are not above being
> children spanked every week. And that's
> exactly why I learn this crap. That's exactly
> why we did better and I think you are fooling
> yourself if you think any other reason. It's
> expected, I can smile at it. I know I wouldn't
> have studied so hard for it unless I had to do
> it. Twenty percent of my grade was on the
> line. And you got to do it for the grades, and
> that's what motivates people!
> —Second-year medical student

Medical education has traditionally held a reputation for a high level of demand on its students, at both the undergraduate and the graduate level. Increased rates of stress, alienation and cynicism among students have been attributed to the process of medical education itself (Becker et al. 1977; Coombs and Boyle 1971; Lloyd and Gartrell 1983; Bloom 1973). Studies that have examined the potential sources of stress within the environment have found perceptions of learning overwhelming amounts of information in too little time (Coombs and Boyle 1971), lack of relevance between curriculum and future roles (Funkenstein 1968), perceived hurdle jumping during the first two years of medical school (Coombs and Boyle 1971), and dealing with unlimited numbers of sick and dying patients in the clinical years (Zoccolillo 1988). One student aptly explained that the frustration she felt in learning the amount of required information in medical school was "like taking a sip from a firehose."

With the belief that medical education is not only content oriented but also a process for socialization into the profession of medicine, concern about the effects which the educational experience has had on student attitudes toward medicine has been a topic of research investigation. Two studies conducted in the 1950s reflected an approach emphasizing that the value of the educational process lay in preparation for or socialization into the profession of medicine. Research conducted at Cornell Medical School by a group of sociologists from Columbia University found that the educational process contained sequential and often stressful events that were essential in helping students frame their perspectives as future physicians.

The tacit knowledge arising as a result of these stressful experiences was critical in helping the student handle future professional concerns, such as uncertainty in clinical decision making (Fox 1989). The experience of working on the cadaver in anatomy helped prepare students to deal with their fear of death. The discomfort which they felt when examining their peers in a physical diagnosis course helped desensitize them to the issues surrounding the human body (Merton 1957).

Becker and sociologists from the University of Chicago conducted a study of student attitudes at the University of Kansas Medical School. Their results (1961), in sharp contrast to the Cornell study, suggested that the educational environment negatively affects student attitudes toward patients. Becker, examining the impact of stress arising from student expectations and existing realities, reported that students respond to conflicting demands of a separate and distant faculty by secretly scapegoating them. Mizrahi (1986), in a study of interns in internal medicine, found a similar situation. Interns responding to the conflict of meeting heavy service demands while providing thorough and complete patient care developed a system called "getting rid of patients" (GROP). The behavior served to maintain the service load at a "reasonable level" while "keeping" only those patients who would provide interesting teaching material for the faculty.

Studies from the Comprehensive Care Program at Cornell suggest that students were treated as future colleagues by the faculty and were able to derive functional professional attitudes from seemingly stressful events. The provocative issue arising from the University of Kansas research is how students "survive" a perceived inhumane educational environment by developing their own social system with an internal logic and rules. Mizrahi's results suggest that this pattern of unrealistic expectations continues into residency and the "survival" response of the house staff interferes with the quality of patient care.

From the two classic studies of Merton and Becker it is clear that students undergo a great deal of stress in their medical training. The profession of medicine, with its consistent confrontation with life-and-death issues and its emotional demand on the physician, is a highly stressful occupation. Whether medical schools as they are presently established provide a process whereby students are systematically confronted with stressors that help them develop appropriate professional values or stressors that set them in opposition to faculty and patients remains to be studied. What is clear is that stressors in medical education are not there by perfect design, established to provide hurdles for the student. Instead these stressors appear to be accidents of history which have, over time, taken on a tradition of professional importance.

The questions addressed by this chapter revolve around innovations of the past few decades and the impact these innovations have had on humanism in medical education. Have they improved the process of student adaptation? Have they significantly added to the student's knowledge base? The final test of any innovation is its end product. Will students exposed to educational innovations become more caring, humanistic physicians?

Traditionally, medical education has been structured in a manner which in some ways defies innovative moves. Such traditions as the "lock step" approach to medical education (two years of basic sciences and two years of clinical sciences), reliance on the lecture method during the first two years, overutilization of house staff as teachers, and reliance on clinical teaching in the tertiary care centers continue to dominate medical education, making major reforms problematic.

Because the structural problems are not only historically based but also heavily burdened with economic underpinnings of private medicine (Starr 1982), most institutions set on medical reform have had to consider the financial implications of change. Indeed, the economics of health care in the United States has a decided impact on the types of innovations chosen and the method by which a medical school goes about reforming itself (Funkenstein 1968). For instance, with the present national move toward a reemphasis of ambulatory care and shortening of hospital stays, medical education institutions have responded by examining the possibilities of clinical training in outpatient departments rather than hospital wards. The role of private funding in medical education innovations is also critical. The Josiah Macy Foundation, the Robert Wood Johnson Foundation, the Commonwealth Fund, the W. K. Kellogg Foundation, and other such groups can take credit for the majority of innovations described here. Their role in formulating what will be innovative and funding what they consider effective and implementable has been indispensable in the history of medical education. The driving commitment of private foundations to medical education is symbolically represented by the Flexner Report of 1910. Funded by the Carnegie Corporation, Abraham Flexner examined the status of medical education at United States institutions. His report signaled the rise of medical education as one of the most serious educational endeavors in the United States. Although funding clearly is central to educational reform, we will not address it further in this chapter. It is clear, however, that most extensive innovations must find favor in the court of some benefactor.

History of Medical Education

Although much praise has gone to Flexner as the major "originator" of contemporary medical education, his report actually solidified an emergent trend initiated at Johns Hopkins twenty years earlier. The lock step approach in medical education and emphasis on basic science research began at the Baltimore medical school. Before Johns Hopkins's curriculum, medical schools varied in their level of competence. Indeed, there were no standard requirements, and many schools had no laboratories, hospitals, or full-time teaching staff. By 1893 sciences such as microbiology were fully advanced areas of academic interest, and Hopkins instituted a structure for medical education that continues to be the paradigm in the United States. Influenced by the German tradition of professionalism (R. Kremmer, personal conversations), medical education was based in a university setting with a full-time faculty and a hospital, where students were required to attend two years of basic science lectures followed by two years of clinical education at the bedside. Many of the Johns Hopkins's faculty members were trained in Germany under the new "ideology of science" with a commitment to teaching science as fundamental to practicing medicine (Morantz-Sanchez 1985). Indeed, Flexner's report, although not contradicting the Hopkins innovation, placed more value on preventive health maintenance, the history of medicine, teaching the scientific method (rather than applying it), and emphasizing the relevance of basic sciences. He condemned didactic lectures as useless and felt the most appropriate teaching modality to be in the clinic (Jonas 1978).

The impetus for accepting Hopkins's approach may well have been as much political as pedagogical. During the early 1900s allopathic medicine was competing with homeopathic medicine, chiropractic medicine, and osteopathy. With the introduction of a scientific basis at a time when discoveries in bacteriology, asepsis, and anesthesia were making allopathic medicine seem somewhat miraculous, the Hopkins model was eagerly adopted (Jonas 1978). What successfully distinguished allopathic medicine from other areas of health care delivery was its connection to the sciences. As a result of the Flexner Report, medical education became standardized in its admissions and course requirements and the American Medical Association's Council on Medical Education and Hospitals introduced minimal requirements for accreditation of U.S. medical schools. The Flexner-inspired reforms were so quickly and uncritically accepted that Flexner's own cautionary words a decade later went unheeded. He raised concern about the move to standardization that resulted in compartmentalization of disciplines and "depressing uniformity" of curricula (Williams 1980). Flexner intended for his suggested reforms to raise the norm of quality education that existed in the United States at the beginning of the twentieth century. Instead, his recommendations had become the unquestioned standard for quality education, and institutions became more rigid in their adaptations and less inventive in their approach to teaching.

The drive to standardize medical education remained entrenched in the United States until the 1950s, when two independent innovations changed the direction of medical education. In 1950, Edward Bridge at the State University of New York at Buffalo initiated a program directed toward improving the learning environment of medical students by teaching teachers to teach. The Buffalo experiment was based on a concern among the faculty that students too quickly lost their original excitement for learning and rapidly resorted to memorization for tests rather than developing skills in critical thinking and reasoning (Miller 1980). In 1952, the Western Reserve University faculty chose as its primary mission to change the educational environment of its medical school along with its curriculum (Williams 1980). Western Reserve had traditionally promoted competition among its students and had created an atmosphere in which the relationship between students and faculty was severely strained. In 1956, results of a near-total revision of Western Reserve's curriculum were actualized when the entering class of medical students became the first participants in what was called an "uncontrolled experiment in medical education." For both institutions, innovations were considered and created out of a basic concern for fostering a humane educational environment for the students. The innovations at Buffalo and Western Reserve set in motion a ripple effect of educational experiments.

With the GPEP Report (AAMC 1984) came a restatement of the Flexner Report, with a renewed emphasis on the process of learning medicine rather than a definition of what was to be learned. Issues such as how one learns, the relevance of what one learns, and the surroundings within which one learns once again were in the spotlight of pedagogical concerns. Yet the GPEP Report came after a major innovative wave had already begun. In Canada in 1969, McMaster University was established with an innovative use of the problem-based approach to learning basic and clinical sciences. McMaster ushered in the present era of experimentations in medical education.

The Theoretical Framework: Review of Innovations in Medical Education

To spotlight the many innovations occurring in the United States, we developed a theoretical model that has the heuristic intent of covering the field in as systematic a manner as possible (see figure). By referring to the

A Model for Classifying Innovations in Medical Education in United States Medical Schools*

FOCUS	LEVEL OF EDUCATIONAL INNOVATION		PROGRAM GOALS
	Course Emphasis	*Institutional Emphasis*	*Attitudes and Behaviors*
Student	Self understanding, orientation programs, mentor programs, peer support	Problem-based learning	Lowered stress levels, increased self esteem
Patient	Programs aimed at understanding the patient/medical ethics, communication skills	Community-oriented education	Increased understanding of psychosocial information, improved doctor-patient relations
Faculty	Competency-based information	Offices of research and faculty development	Increased value of teaching, decreased distance between rewards for teaching
Examples of Curricular Outcomes	Increased number of student support services and courses on patient issues	Increased number of new courses crossing departmental boundaries	Integration of psychosocial information with biotechnological approach

*To read outcomes for organizational and curricular reforms, read down the columns. To read outcomes for student and faculty attitudes and behaviors, read across the rows.

theoretical framework of this chapter we hope to highlight some current innovations while also suggesting the differences among them. The programs we have chosen are ones that we believe exemplify an approach to humane teaching in medical education. Our major area of focus is on the undergraduate curriculum rather than residency training, for the majority of innovations are presently occurring at the medical school level, although this is not to deny the increasing interest in revising house staff training. In addition, our intent has been to cover educational innovations mainly in the United States. Many exciting programs are being developed throughout the world, knowledge of which could advance educational programs in this country. However, we believe that certain cultural and socioeconomic patterns in the United States have had a direct bearing on the amount and type of educational reform occurring here and examining other countries would complicate the analysis.

For purposes of this chapter the types of reforms are best categorized by the course/institutional dichotomy. In addition to the level of innovational change, we also categorized such changes by the particular focus of the innovation. These appeared to fall into three major categories—student-oriented, patient-oriented, and faculty-oriented—as shown in the figure.

The course level reforms are primarily found within departments and are predominantly course structured. At this level, programs addressing the learning needs of the student exemplify the student-oriented programs being developed. Peer support groups and the Balint group (Balint 1972) are examples. We have chosen to examine the current movement toward offering orientation programs and programs that support students' individual coping behaviors through medical school (section I below). Course innovations that focus on patient-centered education fall into the realm of content areas aimed at enhancing the student's understanding of the patient. New content areas in medical education include medical ethics, humanities, and preventive health issues. We examine the present concern about teaching communication skills and the various teaching technologies that have arisen around teaching the doctor-patient relationship in section I. Faculty development courses are exemplified by such trends as that in family medicine programs toward developing faculty skills in research and policy analysis (section IV).

At the institutional level of educational reform, the focus is on the development of total programs within an institution or the redesign of the school's curriculum. Innovations that reflect institutional student-oriented reforms are those programs which have attempted to revise their curricula to make the process of learning more relevant to the student's professional needs. Such student-oriented innovations as the organ system approach at Case Western Reserve University and the alternative curriculum at Rush Medical College are directed at changing the approach to teaching the basic sciences by cutting across departmental lines of authority (section II). Institutional reforms which are seen as patient-oriented fall into the category of teaching within the community or providing early patient contact for students. Schools which provide early experiences with patients or courses taught within the community are considered appropriate for this category. Programs such as Michigan State University's Upper Peninsula program, in which students were to study the basic and clinical sciences within the community, and Case Western Reserve's family clinic, where students follow a family throughout their four years of medical school, are designed to introduce trainees to the primary object of medicine—the patient—early in their education careers (section III). Programs of faculty development arising in an institutional context are those such as the Office of Research in Education at the University of Illinois, which have arisen as a result of the need for educational relevance and reform. In addition, institutional changes that have created a need for faculty to work together across departments, such as faculty development in problem-based Education, serve the function of teaching faculty new interdisciplinary skills (section IV).

Because outcomes are critical in examining the effectiveness of any innovation, we have included possible outcome criteria in the right-hand and lower margins of the figure. Reading down the columns, the outcomes are those which are primarily curricular and institutional.

The figure has a theoretical base. Not only did we attempt to contrast innovations occurring at the course level with those occurring at the institutional level; we also felt that the humane goals of the educational process were attitudinal. We believed that such attitudinal goals were not directly the result of an individual/institutional dichotomy (these were primarily philosophical and pedagogical) but reflected the student/faculty/patient orientation. Drawing from sociological research conducted at Columbia and Chicago, one could interpret the figure in terms of the critique implicit in their analyses. Reading across the rows, the resultant goals are often attitudinal. Reforms that have focused on programs centered on student issues have directed their concerns to creating a better learning environment. The intention is to either help students better understand their own learning needs or bridge the distance between students and faculty. Those innovations that have focused on reinforcing professional attitudes toward the patient have provided more information about patient care issues, such as ethical concerns about biotechnology, or have developed early and sustained clinical contacts for students. The latter programs are often developed with the goal of providing experiences that develop patient-centered values and behaviors.

Unfortunately, examining outcomes of innovation in terms of "humaneness" is a difficult task, one that has rarely been reported. As a result, our task is a descriptive one, using case studies as examples of innovations rather than reporting empirically supported successes. In a way we are offering these case studies as a challenge to the often spoken statement in medical education: "If it isn't broken, don't fix it."

I. Innovations in Course Offerings toward Enhancing Professional Attitudes and Behaviors

Each medical school in the United States has its educational innovators; they tend to cluster within certain departments, rather than being evenly distributed among the faculty, and change radiates out from these groups with pebble-in-the-pond effects throughout the institution. From these leaders come a stream of innovative programs, some of which improve the quality of the students' education, not just the efficiency with which students can gain information or knowledge. Short of restructuring whole segments of the curriculum—as is done in the large problem based learning programs—most of these innovations are courses with "new" subject matter, outlook, or format, offered to supplement, not supplant, the standard curriculum. In this section we look broadly at these courses to see what they can do to humanize the medical curriculum.

New courses are usually viewed from the standpoint of content or structure; it is equally useful to consider, in addition, their intention. Frequently they are aimed at helping the student learn more efficiently. Computer-aided instruction (CAI) initiatives fall into this category. Although much CAI is based upon distinct pedagogic principles such as independent learning and problem solving (particularly with the new interactive discs) its intent remains primarily utilitarian. Courses reflecting computer applications in medical education have developed across the country. Computers are being used to ease the call schedules for house staff (McDaniel 1988), and facilitate and aid applicants and schools on admissions (Paterson 1988). In addition, computer technology has aided the student in self-assessment skills (Willoughby 1988; Thornborough 1988), self-directed learning of the basic sciences (Friedman 1988), and clinical management problems (Durinzi 1988; Hess 1988). Such computer technology also makes it possible for students to work in rural areas, far from the university hospital setting, and continue to receive quality information and computer searches from the university library (Kaufman 1988).

Innovative and creative educational programs also grow out of perceived local need for reform. Particularly since the GPEP Report, close attention has been paid to the process of education as well as to content. It is important to recognize that the structure of medical education is far from value-free and that specific attention must be paid to nurturing the students as well as to "teaching" them. Although the final outcome rests in the quality of care the student provides to patients and—structurally—to society, one can readily hypothesize that the intermediate goals are attitudinal: humble, self-initiating, self-sustaining, gentle, caring, committed students.

Any course aimed at developing humaneness as well as competence must in some way help the student see the patient as a whole person rather than as simply the bearer of disease. Ideally, each patient is cared for (i.e., has an "illness" diagnosed or managed in the context of his or her own life) with respect to occupation, family concerns, and community setting. In order for the physician to recognize the humanness of the patient, the student must know how to have the empathy, affection, and commitment that make caring personal relationships possible. Thus, "humane" innovative programs will fall into two categories. The first are those courses which attempt to more fully teach the students about the humanness of their patients. Courses in communication, geriatrics, AIDS, medical humanities, and ethics all hope to provide the student with information about patients which fits a holistic model. Innovative courses in ethics and in cost containment stand out as being particularly numerous (virtually each month's *Journal of Medical Education* describes one) and necessary. Some of the research which has examined the impact of course offering on the development of values and attitudes in students has focused on changing students attitudes toward AIDS (Farquhar 1988); geriatrics (Van Susteren 1988), and the handicapped (Eminson 1988).

TEACHING COMMUNICATION SKILLS

Courses which teach communication or interviewing skills are neither new nor rare. What has changed within this particular course offering is the increasing variety of experimentation and innovation in the way these courses are devised. Students are provided didactic information on the structure of the interview and are often given suggestions about interviewing such as the use of open-ended questions, active listening skills, etc. Students also have the opportunity to practice interviewing with either real or simulated patients. The simulations can be done by faculty (Bishop 1988), fellow students, or paid actors. The value of simulations is the opportunity for students to come to appreciate psychosocial information with respect to patients as well as an opportunity for patients to provide specific feedback to students regarding their interviewing style and manner of questioning. At the University of Arizona, patient instructors (people with chronic illness who play their illness) are able to provide specific feedback to students, not only about their interviewing style but also concerning the appropriateness of their physical exam and their diagnostic findings. Not only are such student/patient interactions highly reliable in terms of student assessment, they also underscore the value of listening to patients' interests and concerns. To learn from a patient how one's style of interviewing affects them has a powerful impact on developing respect and sensitivity to the patient. Paula Stillman at the University of Massachusetts School of Medicine (Worcester) conducts periodic workshops on how to train patients for simulation and how to develop cases for assessment of student performance as well as for teaching aspects of the exam or the medical interview.

Videotaping is another technology which has increasingly become incorporated into teaching communication and interviewing skills. Students find that viewing tapes of their own performance and critically and carefully examining points of the interview with a faculty member or patient provides a meaningful learning experience. At Dartmouth Medical School, all students in the required primary care clerkship are videotaped interviewing two simulated patients, one at the beginning of the clerkship and one at the end. The cases are developed with psychosocial information as well as hidden agendas. Students are taped interviewing the patient and are observed through a one-way mirror by a faculty person. Simulated patients provide feedback to the students at the end of the interview. All tapes are reviewed before the entire group of clerkship students at the end of the day. By having the "patient" give specific feedback to the student after the interview on the less tangible features of patient care such as whether the patient felt comfortable and cared for, the students are forced to deal quite directly with their patients as people. In addition, by using the tapes for group review, it was found that one could begin on the first day of the clerkship to develop the sense of caring and vulnerability that proves to be so powerful in groups where self-reflection is expected. Not unexpectedly, the faculty also learned much from the videotaping, which provided them with new ideas not only for training but also for sharing innovative techniques with faculty from other departments.

PROGRAMS TO SUPPORT SELF-UNDERSTANDING AND COPING SKILLS

The second category of humane course offerings comprises those aimed at extending humanism to the student. A resurgence of interest in the student's ability to survive medical school may be related to the declining applicant pool, yet the perceived success of those programs aimed at examining the mental health of students point to the ongoing need within medical schools to critically examine how their trainees are treated. Support services have traditionally taken the form of individual counseling for students in academic or personal trouble. Peer support groups and peer tutors have also been offered to students who choose to ask for help. A more recent approach to academic support services for medical students has been the development of programs which prepare entering students for the unique academic rigors of medical school. New orientation programs are being developed across the country which attempt to understand the individual learning needs of the entering students and to offer specific areas of preparation. Schools such as the Medical College of Pennyslvania, Dartmouth Medical School, and Meharry Medical School have used personality assessment inventories such as the Myers-Briggs Personality Type Inventory (Myers 1962) to introduce students to the concept of a personal style of learning, studying, test taking, and time management skills (Shain and Kelliher 1988). Programs which have used the personal study skills approach have developed specific study and note-taking strategies. They have found students often very appreciative and eager to understand. The programs also seem to be effective in the outcome intended. Students do better academically, feel more secure about themselves, and appear to be more willing to ask for help when they are under more stress than they can handle.

The programs are organized so that students are given their personality inventories during orientation. The inventories are then used to demonstrate how people with different learning styles may respond to a variety of lectures, read K-type exam questions, and work in small task-oriented groups such as anatomy labs or small discussion groups such as psychiatry or ethics. Workshops on the personal style and learning strategies are conducted throughout the first and second year of medical school to reinforce the concepts raised during orientation.

Not all schools are using the Myers-Briggs Personality Type Inventory for study skills. Michigan State has organized an extensive prematriculation program for preparing minority students for medical school. Through the use of transactional analysis to understand "life scripts," the program introduces the concept of self-understanding as the major focus of maximizing study skills. In addition, issues such as levels of stress and personal coping styles are examined. Small-group activities are utilized to enhance the concept of interpersonal skills in learning as well as to prepare students for small-group learning experience (Woodbury et al. 1988).

The University of Illinois at Chicago offers an orientation program which takes a holistic approach to introducing medical students to the school. Students are asked to complete a physical stress test during orientation, and specific feedback is provided. In addition, students are encouraged to pursue physical activities as a means of coping with stress. Students are also given an opportunity to work in small-group, problem-based learning tutorials, to encourage an awareness of the various sciences underlying the clinical problems (Nelson and Palmer 1988).

At the University of Maryland an elective six-week prematriculation program is offered for the purpose of preparing students for entering their school. The program continues throughout the year with services offered in academic counseling and peer tutoring for students desirous of help (Willey 1988). The University of Nevada School of Medicine is also providing academic support services to students with the help of personality inventories which they have found helpful for specific feedback and provision of support services (Leiden 1988). The University of Texas at Lubbock offers an elective designed to help students develop self-motivated learning skills. Through the use of the Myers-Briggs Personality Type Inventory students are given specific feedback about their learning style. The course then covers such topics as time management, test-taking skills, creative problem-solving techniques, and critical thinking within a twelve-session course (Gelula and Moore 1988).

It is important to maintain a certain perspective about innovative programs and courses in medical schools. In truth, entering students do not have a very clear sense of medicine's educational failings, of how severely their warmth, empathy, and vulnerability will be strained. When something is done which is strong and new, all that can be hoped is that students will appreciate that someone has done right by them; they will never know how far the programs have come or how innovative they might be. In addition, there is a high probability that most programs will not get recognized or rewarded in professional communities. The bottomline, then, is that the value of what has been done and of what will be done rests in the ownership and enthusiasm more than in the results. The major benefit may well be maintaining the energy of a cadre of embattled innovative medical educators who so badly need the positive reinforcement of success. With each demonstrated improvement, faculty learn how to teach their colleagues to teach better. For it is clearly from a growing pool of skilled teachers rather than from an innovative curriculum that medical education can flourish.

II. Institutional Innovations: Curricular Reforms Emphasizing the Acquisition of Problem-Solving Skills and Clinical Relevance

Innovations defined within an institutional context are those programs which have attempted to change the actual structure of medical education by introducing new methods of teaching which not only challenge traditional approaches but also cut across departmental boundaries. Recently, the move in problem-based learning and community-oriented medical education has resulted in international communication and pedagogical reforms. Rather than focus on the content taught, recent institutional reform has concentrated on the manner in which the information is communicated and as a result schools such as University of New Mexico and Michigan State University have adopted both problem-based learning and community-oriented education. We have chosen to separate community-oriented education and problem-based education because most schools focus more heavily on one or the other. The particular innovations of concern here are those which deal with the student as the object of innovation and are generally refered to as problem-based curricular reform. Such reforms have involved significant programs within one institution, such as Rush Medical College's Alternative Curriculum, or, as in the case of Harvard Medical School and McMaster University, the entire school.

The philosophy behind such innovations is in the humane pedagogical belief that "people are shaped at least as much by how they are treated as by what they are told. . . . In conventional medical education, much of what we do produces in unintended consequences." (Jason 1987) The capacity for effective clinical decision making must be learned, and therefore it is the very process of learning and problem solving that is critical in medicine rather than the content mastered. With the information explosion and increased technological advancements, future physicians must learn to be self-motivated learners and competent problem solvers in order to keep abreast of new information. Curricular reforms such as those described below are also more often found in the United States where attention is more frequently paid to the quality of the curriculum content and increased specialization rather than to the interest of particular health care demands. Two major approaches in institutional innovations have dominated the last several decades of educational reform. One, originating at Western Reserve University in the 1950s, was the curricular revision directed toward integrating the basic sciences into clinical medicine. Focusing on a particular organ system rather than a subject area, the approach was multidepartmental and absorbed traditional boundaries within its approach. The second major innovation began in the 1970s at McMaster University. Termed problem-based learning, its focus has been on teaching basic sciences from clinical patient problems with an emphasis on small-group, self-directed learning. Both innovations attempted to define basic science content within clinical practice and brought the focus away from the theoretical to a more practical and applied approach to the sciences (Barzansky et al. 1983).

ORGAN SYSTEM BASED CURRICULUM

The organ system based curriculum developed at Western Reserve University has been incorporated into various degrees across the country. The intent from Western Reserve University was to offer a "relevant" curriculum for medical education with the information taught around the human body rather than within departmental domains. The hope of the originators was that, by creating an atmosphere of learning rather than competition and organizing the basic sciences around relevant clinical areas rather than theoretical domains, the adversary relationship between students and faculty would diminish. In addition, the grading system was changed to a pass/fail approach (Williams 1980). As a result, the organ system rather than the discipline dominated the teaching. Basic science courses were organized around a particular organ, resulting in such disciplines as anatomy, biochemistry, and physiology, teaching as a team about the cardiovascular or endocrine system as the unit of instruction. The intuitive appeal of the organ system approach was that it was easily translatable into relevance for the profession of medicine. It also brought diverse faculty together to formulate how a content objective would be taught emphasizing the various roles of the basic clinical science areas in medicine.

PROBLEM-BASED LEARNING

The second area of pedagogical reform which has dramatically changed medical education institutionally also carried the banner of relevance and has come to be known as problem-based learning. Although initially established within new, developing schools such as Canada's McMaster University, Mercer, and Michigan State, the problem-based method gained credibility within traditional medical schools by several innovations occurring simultaneously. The intent of this model is to offer a "relevant" curriculum through approaching student learning in a meaningful manner. Relevance in problem-based learning is focused not only on the content learned but also on the process by which one learns. Based on Knowles's theory of adult education (Knowles 1970) called androgogy, problem-based learning entails learner responsibility and self-direction. The basic science content is integrated around clinical problems which are designed to elicit appropriate basic sciences information. The problem-based curriculum is usually taught in small groups of students with one or two tutors who are clinicians and/or basic scientists. The problem-based approach to learning has offered a variety of approaches to teaching students. Many schools have adopted the approach with particular courses, or departments have offered problem-based learning as the method for teaching its discipline. The descriptions offered below are of entire programs offering a specific pedagogical type within different institutions. We have chosen to mainly describe only total programs which are offering a "purist" approach to problem-based learning because they are also the programs invested in testing the effectiveness of problem-based learning.

McMaster University. Originating at McMaster University in 1968, the medical school at the university chose to draw upon what was then seen as a radical approach to teaching basic sciences. With the use of a clinical case, a group of six students and a tutor undertook the task of developing the necessary "learning issues" in the basic sciences in order to teach one another.

As it was originally established, McMaster medical students learned all the basic science information in small tutorial groups. With cases designed to elicit questions about the basic sciences areas students were then expected to list the basic sciences questions and pursue an answer. The tutors were there to help guide the learning but not to offer didactic information. As a new school McMaster was able to hire faculty interested in this innovation and resistance which is commonly seen toward innovations was not found at McMaster. People such as Howard Barrows, a neurologist interested in clinical problem solving, joined the faculty with a desire to develop simulated problems in order to teach the problem-solving process in clinical decision making. As a result, the school took a giant step toward innovation, taking the teaching out of the hands of the faculty and putting it on the shoulders of the student with guidance and encouragement. The role of the faculty became that of stimulating the student's desire to learn the information. The intent was to help develop better problem solvers and critical thinkers rather than merely encourage memorization and recall. The technology which developed at McMaster's problem-based curriculum has been used and modified throughout the world. Such techniques as the standardized patient (a person trained to simulate a clinical problem) (Barrows 1976), the focused problem (a clinical problem specifically designed to encourage questions in specific areas of basic and clinical science) (Brazeau et al. 1987), and the triple jump (an assessment procedure which examines students' interviewing skills and hypotheses generation) (Kaufman 1985) were incorporated into other schools' curricula regardless of whether they were problem based.

Student assessment was also developed to be consistent with the philosophy of student-directed learning. Students were assessed on their ability to develop and test hypotheses rather than pass a content exam. What McMaster provided was not only a new approach to teaching medical students; it also offered the world of medical education an opportunity to examine its traditional curriculum and experiment with new technologies.

Michigan State University. A new preclinical program was established in 1964 at Michigan State University which was called the College of Human Medicine (CHM). Its original planning committee developed educational goals which were designed to provide innovative teaching and individualized student programs enhance self-direction and self-evaluation skills, and offer a community orientation.

In 1968 twenty-seven students were admitted into the preclinical program. By 1972, a degree-granting curriculum came into place called track I. Within three years of starting the curriculum the Michigan State faculty chose to incorporate problem-based learning with focal problems as a format for teaching its students. An innovative, focused problem track, track II, was therefore introduced shortly after track I's inception. The track II curriculum came about largely as a result of thirteen students requesting an entirely problem-based curriculum after their initial problem-based experience in phase one. With the aid of designated faculty and the dean of the medical school, focused problems were developed to aid the students in learning the basic science content within student-directed small groups.

Concern about the curriculum grew among faculty when institutionalizing of track II became imminent. Major compromise was the strategy for maintaining its existence. Such compromises as the same required content in both tracks as well as content-based student assessment were seen as necessary to program continuation but "detrimental to the original ideas of problem-based learning." As one of the directors indicated: "Patient care has lost its central role as a stimulus for learning, having been replaced by the concept list. The discovery method of learning has declined, as the faculty has defined the content to be learned in more and more detail. Student directed learning has lost out" (Brazeau et al. 1987).

The existence of two tracks allowed Michigan State to compare the effectiveness of two different learning experiences. The results, which would be echoed by other schools examining problem-based learning with traditional teaching modalities, was that there were few differences between the two in such traditional outcomes as national boards, standardized tests, clerkship performances, etc. Results in specialty choice, however, suggested that students in track I chose more subspecialties while track II students more frequently chose areas of family medicine, psychiatry, and pediatrics. Student-directed, problem-based learning was as effective as the traditional lecture in teaching students content in the basic sciences.

University of New Mexico. In New Mexico, the decision was made to incorporate both problem-based learning and community-oriented teaching appropriate for the geographical area of the country. The University of New Mexico has been established with a mission to meet the medical needs of the highly rural state, and by the early 1970s was found to be unsuccessful at meeting the manpower needs for the state. Program developers looked for an approach that would help motivate students to enter rural primary care. They had taught a course in primary care for students within the traditional curriculum and found it to be unsuccessful at influencing attitudes and behavior. As a result the directors decided to develop an entire curriculum which would be oriented toward preparing students for entering rural primary care. Examining the programs at McMaster and Michigan State, they felt that problem-based, self-motivated learning with an intensive community experience would prepare and encourage students to pursue primary care. In addition they felt that relevance of basic science information would be more meaningful to students, thereby providing a more humane approach to medical education.

The University of New Mexico was an already established medical school and the choice of such innovation required outside funding. In addition, because they offered a major innovation alongside a traditional program, resistance to change from within was great and required the new program, the primary care curriculum (PCC), to "prove its effectiveness" where tradition had guaranteed the success of the other. As a result, New Mexico, receiving funding from the Kellogg Foundation, set itself up as an experimental program within an ongoing traditional curriculum (Kaufman 1985).

With a group of ten, then fifteen, and finally twenty of the seventy-five yearly matriculating students at New Mexico, PCC quickly ensured its success by student interest. Students learn the basic sciences in small tutorial groups with problem-focused cases. During the summer of the first year all students enter a rural New Mexico community to spend four months with a primary care physician. They return to campus, resume small groups, and upon successful completion of National Boards of Medical Examiners I, enter the third year along with their classmates in the traditional curriculum. Research from New Mexico's program found that students did as well academically as did those in the traditional curriculum (Moore-West and O'Donnell 1985). In addition, PCC students reported less stress in their learning environment and found their curriculum to be more supportive and relevant than did students from the conventional track. (Moore-West 1986). The results were a surprise to the program directors because of the high ambiguity within PCC's curriculum and the attitude in the school that problem-based learning would not be appropriate for the average New Mexico student. Such results support the observation in Becker's early research that there is a powerful relationship between how one is taught and professional self-esteem. As at Michigan State University, students graduating from the primary care curriculum were more likely to sustain their original interest in primary care fields than students in the traditional curriculum (Moore-West and O'Donnell 1985; Schmidt et al. 1987; Mennin et al. 1987). Another important finding coming from New Mexico was the profound impact which the existence of curricular innovation had on traditional education. Although a problem-based curriculum has developed during the clerkship years with an increased emphasis on community-oriented health care (Kaufman 1988), the traditional curriculum has made equal strides by incorporating small-group, problem-based learning into its curriculum along with computer instruction modules. As a result of PCC's existence, self-reflection and educational experimentation have become an ongoing element in the medical school as a whole; New Mexico no longer has a traditional curriculum but two dynamic evolving approaches to teaching students. In the summer of 1986, the faculty of the University of New Mexico School of Medicine agreed to continue PCC. Although it could only prove itself equally as effective as traditional education as measured by student performance on content outcomes such as NBME I and Clerkship Performance, the faculty agreed that the continued existence of PCC offered an atmosphere of pedagogical change and dynamic experimentation which had become irresistible.

Rush Medical College. In 1984 Rush piloted a program called the alternative curriculum which was an alternative to the traditional two-year preclinical curriculum. The alternative curriculum is a small-group, problem-focused format. Rush differs from the preceding schools in its rationale for paying attention to the problem-based curricular structure. It is a private school which is not as interested in primary care needs for the state as in providing quality curriculum for its students. The decision to choose a problem-based approach to curriculum development came from the dean's office and medical student programs who were interested in quality education and faculty development. Money used to pay outside schools to provide basic science education to Rush students was turned back to the school for the development of the alternative curriculum. Rush developed a curriculum which could rely on clinicians to teach basic sciences as small-group tutors. This was a strategic decision because of limited basic science resources as well as the interest in modeling clinical decision making. The decision also set a precedent for allowing the basic sciences to be taught by clinicians who are not expert in the field. As a result of limited basic science faculty, Rush's alternative curriculum developed guidebooks for students which provided both case objectives and various available learning exercises to facilitate their learning basic science content (Gotterer et al. 1987).

At Rush students learn the sciences basic to medicine in small-group tutorials which are supplemented by scheduled sessions with resource faculty. The latter sessions provide students an opportunity to ask questions as well as seek specific assistance with problems for which they perceive a need for help.

As with other schools with two curricula, Rush has recently evaluated the effectiveness of both approaches. Unlike the previous two longitudinal evaluations, the evaluation comparing the two curricula was carefully conducted by a group of school evaluators rather than evaluators salaried by the innovative programs. Very preliminary results indicate that there are few differences between the tracks on such performance outcomes as NBME I, course performance, and clerkship rotation evaluations. Interestingly, results in such areas as attitudes and clinical decision making also indicated few differences. Yet, the very presence of the alternative curriculum at Rush has resulted in a type of Hawthorne Effect. Along with the introduction of an innovative curriculum has come a process of self-reflection and critique within the traditional curriculum. The resultant changes have complicated any "objective" measures of program outcomes; yet such changes have had an undeniably positive impact on student learning experiences.

Harvard University. The first class of students to enter Harvard's Oliver Wendell Holmes Society entered in 1985. Thus Harvard's innovation in problem-based learning has only begun. As elsewhere, students involved in the innovative curriculum were self-selected. The society is the beginning of Harvard's "new pathway" to educating its students for medicine.

Students learn the sciences basic to medicine in problem-based tutorial groups. Three to five lectures weekly address current issues in the basic sciences. In addition, a longitudinal session on the patient/doctor relationship runs throughout the four years with an afternoon a week devoted to interviewing, ethics, communication, etc. This program will also continue the problem-based approach into the clerkship years, providing a continuity not previously seen in problem-based learning (Ramos and Moore 1987).

Dartmouth Medical School. Such a combination as Harvard's is an approach to problem-based innovation which may be attractive to many schools across the country, because it is less threatening to departmental autonomy. By combining both methods of teaching—the traditional lecture and the innovative small-group tutorial—schools which would shy away from total structural revision might consider a more modified approach to incorporating innovations such as problem-based learning. At Dartmouth Medical School the approach of combining lectures and small problem-based tutorials has been under way since 1980. The course Health, Society, and the Physician (HSP) is required for fourth-year students. Developed by the Department of Community and Family Medicine, it offers lectures, problem-based small groups, and thoroughly developed and continually revised resource manuals to teach the psychosocial, economic, and ethical bases of medicine at a point in the curriculum when they are relevant to the student (fourth year). Faculty from all over the college are recruited to tutor in the small groups. Due to the uniqueness of this approach to teaching, faculty are provided extensive information on the cases used in small groups as well as training in problem-focused, student-directed learning. The HSP directors have dealt with the challenge of organizing lecture content to easily interface with small-group learning and have opted to place the emphasis on the focused problems rather than the content-directed lecture. Students and faculty involved in HSP continually ask for more experiences, and Dartmouth is presently considering the option of combining lectures and small problem-focused groups to teach areas other than psychosocial information (Colby et al. 1986).

Other medical schools' innovations. Across the country schools are developing alternative curricula with problem-based format. Bowman Gray Medical School in North Carolina has developed an alternative curriculum called the parallel curriculum, which has been operating for a year. The program directors report the program as highly successful. The initial objectives for initiating problem-based learning are based on an ongoing interest from the school faculty for improving student education. The specific institutional outcomes the directors hope to achieve are a rejuvenation of faculty enthusiasm and interest in educating physicians-to-be, the modeling of educational practices and philosophies as a "living laboratory," the nurturing of potential clinical scientists among the students, and the development and refinement of techniques for scientific educational research (personal conversations; also Wofford 1987). As at schools preceding Bowman Gray, the very initiation of a new program has provoked faculty self-examination and encouraged curricular reform. Ten years ago, when New Mexico initiated problem-based learning, the directors were concerned that students would not select the primary care curriculum because they knew nothing about problem-based learning. Today, problem-based learning has become so well known that students are choosing Bowman Gray over other North Carolina schools because of its alternative curriculum. The early concerns about the appropriateness of problem-based learning within medical education have been alleviated. Results point to comparable academic performances by students in traditional and innovative curricula, and there is some suggestion that students in the innovative programs are less distressed.

Southern Illinois Uuniversity will begin a problem-based track in 1989. Schools such as Dartmouth Medical School, Tufts, and the University of Colorado have developed problem-based learning within individual teaching departments. The American Association of Medical Colleges has expressed a commitment to problem-based learning in funding various interested schools to visit medical schools with specific problem-based innovations.

The existence of problem-based learning has provided a stimulus for curricular experimentation and change. Like its predecessor, the organ-system curriculum, the innovation has created another opportunity for traditional medical education to examine itself. Its presence has created a tension within most schools of medicine to examine their mission and their approach to meeting their goals. Ultimately, the goal of most medical schools is toward creating a humane, competent physician who can provide quality health care. Problem-based learning has reintroduced the concept of examining the process of learning along with the content being taught toward meeting that goal. When the process of learning was examined at the University of New Mexico, students in problem-based learning were far less stressed than their colleagues. Such results suggest that when schools look to change how they teach, they enter into a relationship with their students that is far more humble and collegial than when they are concerned merely with what they teach.

III. Institutional Innovations: Emphasizing Continuity of Care and Community-Based Learning Experiences

In the early twentieth century, predominantly influenced by the Johns Hopkins model of education, the site for teaching clinical medicine moved from ambulatory care apprenticeships to the wards and specialty clinics of teaching hospitals. Now it may be returning to community-based ambulatory settings. Three models presently dominate the approach to teaching in the community. One approach offers students an opportunity to work with patients early in their educational career in order to place the basic sciences they are learning into a meaningful perspective. Students will work with community faculty or preceptors in a variety of specialities for a month or six-week rotation or will "follow" a clinical preceptor over a semester or year's duration. The latter approach is physician centered. A second approach which is more patient centered offers students an opportunity to extend their training into the community or work in ambulatory care clerkships. The latter approach suggests that clinical medicine should be taught outside the hospital wards in order to provide students with appropriate training for their future in medicine. The movement appropriately termed "the ambulatory care movement" is rapidly gaining attention among many schools as an appropriate site for learning clinical medicine. The third model, termed community-oriented primary care, not only teaches clinical medicine in the community, but suggests that the community may be the patient itself, rather than the individuals living within its geographical boundaries. Students are encouraged to work with preceptors as well as community leaders and agency directors in order to understand and help treat the community's health problem, which may be creating medical concerns for the citizens.

Teaching in the ambulatory care setting or within the community itself is not a new concept, but its recent popularity may be as much driven by economic incentives as by pedagogical concerns. The economic factors are shortened hospital stays, less willingness of insurers to pay for education-related expenses, and competition between teaching and clinical care for expensive subspecialists' time in medical centers. With the advent of DRGs, patients are in the hospital too briefly for students to see, much less manage, all but a small part of the evolution of an illness.

Fortunately, these economic forces may result in medical education moving toward more humanistic ends. To learn medicine in an ambulatory care setting provides students an opportunity to deal with patients and their families in a comprehensive and longitudinal manner not possible in a tertiary care setting. The opportunity to see patients over time provides the basis and rationale for learning communication skills and appreciating the need for understanding the psychosocial needs of the patient. What motivates one patient to change his or her behavior, another to prevent an illness from occurring, and still others to not seek help are critical questions in understanding health care behavior, and important in providing quality medical care to patients. This section explores the impact of changes in the structure of patient care and how these changes might affect humanism in medical education.

The patient's health care environment has changed substantially in the last thirty years. Two-week hospitalizations for parturition and three weeks for myocardial infarctions have been reduced to stays lasting hours or days. Thirty years ago patients were seen by students in subspecialty clinics, emergency rooms, hospital wards on the staff service, or occasionally private offices. Now it is becoming increasingly common for these same patients to encounter a medical student on a home visit (with a physician, visiting nurse, or new health practitioner), in an immediate care center, or in the office of a community physician, in addition to the previous settings. This change in the environment of medical education creates a major opportunity for the teaching of humane values that place the patient and family, rather than the disease or organ system, at the center of care.

In ambulatory settings students can potentially observe and participate in physician/patient relationships that emphasize continuity of care. In the past, knowing the patient for a three-week hospitalization for a myocardial infarction was the best continuity experience medical education could offer, but such hospitalizations center on the disease and the patient's survival. This cannot compare in terms of patient-centeredness with knowing the patient for the time after discharge when he or she is readjusting goals and functional status to face a new reality. We need new models that develop the potential for ambulatory continuity. In accommodating to the economic realities of the 1990s and following patients in ambulatory setings, substantial advantages for humanism in medical education may result. Knowledge of the patient will go beyond the immediate biomedical and coping factors. In the ambulatory setting patients maintain more control and are participants rather than passive recipients of care. And care is more likely to be provided in the context of the patient's whole life, with attention to family, work, and community.

The historical shift of medical education toward patient- rather than disease-centered learning began with the development of the family clinic program at Western Reserve School of Medicine in the middle 1950s (Kennell et al. 1961). Selected pregnant women were offered the chance to be followed by medical students from middle pregnancy through the first one or two years of their children's lives. Over the next ten years preceptorship programs (usually elective) began to appear in which students could work in a physician's office, developing a relationship with both the physician and the patients. Currently, at least 70 of the 127 medical schools in the country offer some version as an elective (Dietrich et al. 1986).

Longitudinal electives have been described from many medical schools. They are typically based in the Department of Family Practice and usually involve students in the preclinical years, periodically spending ambulatory care time (often a half day every one or two weeks) with community physicians. Student roles vary from being an observer to being a closely supervised provider of care. Some programs emphasize the student getting to know some patients and families very well and doing home visits. McGann at Stanford had students do one family study, a detailed exploration and analysis of family structure of one patient whom students followed in the context of a preclinical preceptorship in primary care (Nutting 1987).

EARLY SUSTAINED CLINICAL CONTACT

An example of community preceptorships will serve to elaborate on this general model of teaching in the community and show the potential for accommodation to many institutional situations. The Department of Community and Family Medicine, Dartmouth Medical School, has provided a longitudinal preceptorship called the family medicine longitudinal elective (FMLE) for its preclinical students for almost ten years. Students are assigned to a community family physician and are expected to spend two to four half days a month of elective time with the physician during the first and second years of medical school. The program began small and was initially directed at students with a strong interest in family practice. At first approximately ten students (15 percent) from each class participated annually, with many students being turned down due to lack of nearby family practices suitable for teaching. A supplemental curriculum was provided in which students met in a seminar format for 1.5 hours monthly to discuss particular patients or topics of interest with course faculty. Many students developed a small cadre of patients whom they knew well over time, but some did not. Some students became active participants in care (interviewing patients, collecting vital signs, discussing management options with the patient and supervising physician) while others remained strictly observers.

A change in the program's philosophy led to two major changes in it about three years ago. The change was toward making the program more available to everyone rather than just to the most highly motivated students. Initially, the pool of community family physicians was greatly expanded by enlarging the geographic region that was considered. If an excellent preceptor was available 90 minutes away, students were allowed to go if they wanted to, even if that meant being there for shorter periods of time. Student participation soon exceeded 50 percent of each class, but, as expected, the dropout rate rose. Also students were presumably less motivated, found the distances more formidable than they had expected, or found the demands of the required curriculum greater than they initially thought.

To face these problems but still accommodate student demand, a second modification was made. A new component was added to the required curriculum called the clinical interaction (CI). In this experience, *all* students are expected to have four interactions over the course of the first year of medical school, following a clinical preceptor or a patient or family experiencing high impact illness (pregnancy, nursing home placement). Experienced clinicians drawn from a range of specialities (primary care physician and medical surgical subspecialties) supervise one or two students each. Not all these student/patient relationships work out in a longitudinal sense (the student is unable to follow a patient or family over time), in which case the student fulfills the four interaction requirement by observing the preceptor with a range of patients. As an alternative, the more highly motivated students still can opt for the family medicine longitudinal elective as a way of meeting their clinical interaction requirement. More students now have the ongoing experience with a patient. Fewer students drop out and, in fact, more "drop in," that is, switch to the family medicine longitudinal elective during the course of the year because they find they want a more intensive relationship than clinical interaction can provide. Thus at one school with limited community teaching resources, the preclinical longitudinal preceptorship model has been adopted to meet student demand and still provide high-quality longitudinal experiences that teach a humane perspective by centering on individual physicians in their interactions with patients.

New Mexico's approach to offering first-year students early clinical experiences was a model similar to that at Dartmouth Medical School. In addition, the primary care curriculum offered its own early and extended community preceptorship, phase IB. Phase IB is a four-month experience in rural communities of New Mexico for students completing their first year of medical school. During their IB experience, students work with a primary care physician. In addition they are expected to develop a research or service project designed to help the community itself. Although students are expected to apply problem-based learning by integrating the basic sciences with the clinical problems they are seeing, they are also expected to apply sociocultural/environmental sciences to the communities in which they work. To prepare students for this experience, the problems developed for students prior to their IB experience are heavily weighted with both psychosocial and cultural factors. The emphasis for the IB experience is to promote an attitude of responsibility toward both individual patients and communities for the development of adequate health promotion and illness prevention (Voorhees et al. 1985).

Outcomes of such programs are usually measured in terms of satisfaction. Students like them. Faculty members do, too, and that is essential since they are usually volunteers. Patients seem to like them also. Measuring outcome beyond satisfaction is a formidable task. Harris failed to find any impact on career choice (Harris et al. 1982; Harris and Effert 1983). However, expectations about outcomes must be kept in perspective. These longitudinal elective experiences generally can be measured in terms of less than one hundred hours total and should be seen in the context of many thousands of hours of medical school education. How much impact can we expect? The difficulty of identifying adequate control groups and obtaining study groups of sufficient size to have the power to detect differences in relevant outcomes, even if we know exactly what differences we hope to achieve, is problematic. Although careful evaluations are crucial, lack of rigorous outcome results at this time do not justify ignoring the descriptive outcomes.

AMBULATORY CARE, COMMUNITY-ORIENTED CLERKSHIPS

Like many schools, Dartmouth Medical School has a required ambulatory care clerkship, the primary care clerkship, which is community based. Because Dartmouth is located in a rural region, all third- or fourth-year students work with community primary care physicians and still have access to the weekly academic curriculum taught at the medical school. The first clerkship director's interests in health promotion created an opportunity to expand the "core curriculum" by focusing on smoking cessation and alcoholism. The director utilized the novel technique of recruiting smokers in the community into a "stop smoking clinic" run by the clerkship students themselves. The apprenticeship component of the clerkship—with students working in the offices of private community physicians—was later supported with explicit goals and objectives, frequent site visits, and preceptor workshops designed to train the community physician as the primary teacher in the clerkship. In addition the recent director established a Balint group modeled after the groups described by the British psychoanalyst Michael Balint to discuss problem patients. It has been the intent of the modified Balint groups to help students examine themselves in relationship to their patients (Balint 1972).

To turn toward more teaching in ambulatory care settings, programs will be required to expand their training facilities and to offer more house staff training within the clinic-based setting. The majority of programs which have used ambulatory care facilities have generally offered a model for primary care intervention. Internal medicine's role within ambulatory teaching sites may be different. Early programs in internal medicine and ambulatory care have directed attention to how best to teach the various subspecialties. A recent survey by O'Donnell (1988) assessing the various programs which teach oncology/hematology in an ambulatory care setting found that 50 percent of the programs have actually developed an ambulatory approach to teaching, but most did not require this.

COMMMUNITY-ORIENTED PRIMARY CARE

A new development that has relevance for the impact of the patient's environment on medical education is community-oriented primary care (Nutting 1987), in which patients are cared for in the context of their community. In a sense the community becomes the patient and the physician makes a commitment to follow and respond to the health status of the community as determined by various measures just as physicians respond to a single patient's vital signs. This is denominator- not numerator-based medicine. Although the concept is new and few programs have experimented with community-oriented primary care programmatically, the Kellogg Foundation has agreed to grant ten demonstration programs an opportunity to develop the concept within medical education.

In 1979, a group of educational institutions in health care training, which mainly train students in community-oriented learning environments, formed an organization called the Network of Community-Oriented Educational Institutions for the Health Sciences. Although generally comprised of third-world countries' medical schools that are new and where community health care is critically needed, the network also has institutions from the United States and other industrialized countries such as Sweden, Denmark, and Great Britain. Currently co-sponsored by the World Health Organization and the Rockefeller Foundation, the network conducts conferences and workshops and acts as an umbrella organization for educational institutions in problem-based and community-oriented medical education. The network's goals are strengthening of membership institutions in their realization of community orientation and problem based learning; strengthening of individual faculty capacities related to community orientation and problem-based learning; development of technologies, approaches, methodologies, and tools appropriate to a community-oriented and problem-based educational system; promoting and coordinating the population-based concepts in the health services system and the educational program; and assisting institutions in countries that have made a political decision to introduce innovations in the training of health personnel (Kantrowitz and Kaufman 1985).

Current and anticipated trends toward shifting more patient care activities to ambulatory care settings will create expanded opportunities for students to learn in more humanistic settings that emphasize continuity of care and management of the patient's health care in the context of the rest of their lives. Such an approach crosses traditional departmental boundaries in its focus on teaching around the patient and puts basic science concepts into humanistic perspective. Many schools have already taken advantage of these opportunities by instituting required and elective preceptorships in the first two years of medical school. Various models have evolved, however, and the next agenda item may be to conduct a more vigorous evaluation of teaching in the clinic and whether the humanistic objectives are being met.

IV. Faculty Development and Educational Innovation

As a movement in its own right, faculty development began in the early 1950s as an experiment in teaching teachers how to teach. The thrust for examining teachers' skills arose from a concern about the process of medical education where students all too quickly lose their initial enthusiasm for learning and rely on their ability to memorize in order to pass exams. The question which arose at the State University of New York at Buffalo was not one of concern about the ability of the student admitted to medical school. Instead, the concern arose from a commitment to improve the learning environment for medical trainees. Buffalo's answer created a movement that has come to be referred to as faculty development. The model intervention was established in the belief that faculty needed training in education in order to be more effective educators/teachers. Implied in this movement of teaching the art of teaching is enhancing the relationship between student and teacher and patient and physician.

With the Buffalo experiment in 1952, faculty development began as an attempt to improve the learning environment for students through improving faculty teaching skills. The 1950s were a time of experimentation and formulation for the approaches in faculty development. Western Reserve and the University of Pennsylvania were independently developing their own approaches to training their faculty which were tied to the institutional climate of the particular medical school itself. The experiment at Buffalo continued to evolve until late in 1958–59 when it became a national workshop series sponsored by the AAMC, the Summer Institute on Medical Teaching. The move toward institutionalization of programs continued into the 1960s when George Miller established the Office of Research in Medical Education at the University of Illinois. Hilliard Jason established the Office of Medical Education and Research Development at Michigan State University and Stephen Abrahamson developed the Division of Research in Medical Education at the University of Southern California. Miller was interested in student assessment, Jason was concerned about problem solving and clinical decision making, and Abrahamson was instrumental in experimenting with various modes of educational technologies for teaching and for student assessment. In addition to the individual institutional offices in medical education, the AAMC also established a section of medical education research called Research in Medical Education (RIME).

By the 1970s substantial research was being published from the three large divisions on medical research and education and people were being trained in research and faculty development. Seventy programs in medical education research were established across the country. With the advent of problem-based learning, schools which were developing educational programs in this method also took responsibility for teaching faculty how to tutor in small problem-based groups.

Faculty development took another turn in the 1970s with the introduction of family medicine as an academic specialty. In addition to the established programs in medical education and research, the need for developing competencies both within the profession as clinicians and among physicians as teachers has given rise to a new trend in faculty education. Specialty-oriented programs in faculty development are being established in the 1980s to ensure a certain level of competency in areas which were previously taken for granted.

The events which occurred around faculty development since the 1950s are important enough to warrant a more detailed history. Most of the innovations in faculty development presently being put forth are actually rediscoveries or derivations of old innovations that were developed in the 1950s. Usually the lack of funding or the high cost in manpower led to many of the programs in faculty development being discontinued or modified. Rarely were the innovations not worthy of continuation, and some are yet to be equalled.

ORIGIN OF FACULTY DEVELOPMENT: CASE STUDY OF BUFFALO EXPERIMENT

The concept of faculty development first became a reality at Buffalo in 1950 under the direction of Edward Bridge. Bridge was concerned with the difficulty which students, arriving at medical school eager to learn and strongly motivated, had with the large amount of material and fast pace in the first year of medical school. He felt that they were too quickly overwhelmed and confused by the necessity to memorize for instant recall without much need for reasoning, thinking, or evaluating (Bridge 1959).

The objectives of Bridge's first seminar on medical education were to provide opportunities for the students to talk without inhibitions regarding themselves, their interests, and the medical curriculum, and to expose the students to a variety of experiences illustrating the human and social aspects of disease (Miller 1980). Due to the seminar objectives, it was decided that the students would meet in small groups with a tutor to maximize discussion around the topics of student concern as well as the pyschosocial content. The seminar began with students meeting in small groups with a clinician tutor for almost two hours every two weeks and with the tutors meeting with each other on the alternate weeks. This continued without interruption for five years and ultimately involved nearly one hundred medical school faculty. After the first six months the focus of the meetings between faculty and students evolved to include encounters with patients and practitioners, visits to hospitals and physicians' offices, and observation of surgical and obstetrical procedures. Despite opposition to this innovation, the seminar faculty were persistent in their conviction that the work of medicine was to deal with people and not with medical content alone (Bridge 1959).

In 1951–52 the pilot program, now called Introduction to Medicine, was expanded to allow the tutors to follow their students into the second year and a new group of tutors was recruited for the entering freshmen. George Miller, a junior faculty member, was chosen to organize the freshman program. Reports of successful and unsuccessful meetings wth students, debates of institutional organization and policies, curriculum organization, and examination techniques were discussed. Bridge introduced into the seminars presentations by experts on such topics as student selection, student study habits, the nature of learning, and the use and abuse of laboratory learning. These experts were professors of education, sociology, psychology, and English; the dean of liberal arts and the dean of education; a social worker; the president of a state teachers' college; and the university director of admissions.

Pivotal in the evolution of the Buffalo experience was an additional faculty series of ten two-hour seminars entitled Adventure in Pedagogy presented by Nathaniel Cantor, an educational anthropologist. He maintained a strong pedagogical approach to learning which enabled the participants to view teaching in an entirely different way. The challenge of the teaching task was to develop strategies in helping the student desire to know what the faculty wanted them to know. Learning and knowledge were not to be seen as equivalent. The basic responsibility of a teacher was to respect rather than judge the student, encouraging a desire to learn rather than to know (Miller 1980).

As a result of what the participants felt was a positive experience, a new project was conceived for the next five years. This one-year project was for four Buffalo faculty and four visiting faculty to do an initial two weeks of daily seminars on educational topics and the teaching/learning process followed by half of each day throughout the remainder of the year devoted to independent study or seminar discussion of issues in education. The project's four objectives were: (1) determine the importance to the education of medical students of an increased awareness among medical teachers of fundamental educational principles, (2) determine the feasibility of a continuing cooperative effort between a school of medicine and other university divisions in the development of more effective teachers in medicine, (3) assess the effect of changes in mode of instruction that may result from this teacher training program upon medical student learning, and (4) determine the practicality of such an approach to the educational problems of medical schools.

Evaluation of the pilot project was carried out by the Buffalo Educational Research Center under Abrahamson's direction. The hypothesis to be tested was that an increased awareness of educational principles would lead to changes in the attitudes of medical teachers toward the process of medical education and to changes in their institutional educational practices. It was assumed that these attitudinal changes would result in more efficient student learning, so that the instructional changes would lead to more positive attitudes among students toward their own responsibilities, and that these changes would produce medical school graduates better prepared to function as physicians (Miller 1980).

The first round of the Buffalo project occurred in 1956–57 and was remarkably successful. Attitudinal data collected by Rosinski revealed an increased awareness of the variety of techniques available to facilitate the teaching/learning process, a concern for the appropriateness of techniques used, increased awareness of the purposes of medical education, increased awareness of the importance of defining objectives, increased appreciation of the role of basic scientists by clinicians and vice versa, increased willingness to explore and to accept alternate views about educational content and process, enhanced appreciation of the contribution to medical education that could be made by professional educators, increased awareness of the complexities of formal education and the learning/teaching process, and recognition that knowledge of a subject is an insufficient criterion for the preparation and identification of a good teacher (Miller 1980).

By 1958, due to diminished interest among the faculty, the program changed form into an intensive two-week residential program with each of the general themes explored in the full year to be included. Those elements that had proved the most informative and provocative were included. With American Association of Medical Colleges sponsorship, the first summer institute occurred in 1959 with twenty-five participants representing twenty-five medical schools and was an unqualified success. All thought that the experience would influence their teaching. The experience was offered for four years, and 155 faculty members from 56 medical schools in the United States and Canada participated. Two significant research studies directly evolved out of the Buffalo project: Edwin Rosinski's study of the modification of faculty attitudes toward education in medicine and Hilliard Jason's study of teaching practices (Miller 1980).

INDEPENDENT DEVELOPMENTS

Independent of the colonization movements by Buffalo participants, Western Reserve University in 1959 became the site of curriculum innovation which was much discussed, debated, and imitated throughout the United States. Joseph Wearn, dean since 1945, invited Thomas Hale Ham, a respected internist, productive investigator, and gifted teacher at Harvard, in 1950 to be chairman of a faculty committee whose responsibility was to select and define educational objectives, evaluate educational programs, and recommend instructional changes. Two guiding principles aided Ham during the eight years that he held the post: a need for a steadfast spirit of inquiry and rigorous study into the soundness of what was proposed for the educational programs, and the unfailing reminder that students were the central focus around which educational programs were built. In 1956 the Committee on Medical Education proposed an independent Division of Research in Medical Education (RIME), and in 1958 it was established with Ham as its first director. The major research and development focus was education for problem solving in medici.ze (Miller 1980).

At the same time at the University of Pennsylvania, Julius Comroe, chairman of the Departments of Physiology and Pharmacology, set up an informal program designed to improve the quality of faculty lectures and to provide his graduate students guidance in how to use instructional techniques (Camroe 1953). The format he selected would now be called micro-teaching. Each faculty volunteer prepared a fifteen-minute lecture, which was delivered to peers who discussed the volunteer's performance while the volunteer listened to a tape of the lecture. The speaker then rejoined the group and shared with the group a personal analysis of his or her own lecture, which was followed by reactions, comments, criticisms, and praise from the others. The group identified aspects that needed improvement and made a written record of these recommendations for a point of reference for the next round. It wasn't until 1977 that Comroe acknowledged the possibility that professionals from the discipline of education might make a helpful contribution to such efforts (Miller 1980).

In a manner not unlike that at the University of Pennsylvania, Alexander Robertson, who established the Department of Social and Preventive Medicine at the University of Saskatchewan in 1958, labored to establish a curriculum that required active student participation and to provide teachers wtih guidance in the skillful use of instructional methods that would foster such activity. Small-group sessions were selected to fulfill the first goal of active student participation in curriculum planning. The second goal was accomplished through independent observational analysis by a physician and a professional educator of what actually took place in the classroom. Each classroom session observed was taped and the tape replayed the following day to provide objective data for the critique conducted with all departmental teaching faculty members present. Teacher performance was analyzed and evaluated against objectives, pedagogic weaknesses, and strengths. Robertson (1960) reported that "it is only by such rigorous self-evaluation that a group of medical teachers can maintain their teaching skills in the same way as they would wish to maintain their practicing and scientific skills: i.e., by a process of continuing education about education itself."

DIRECT DISSEMINATION OF THE BUFFALO EXPERIMENT

Three personalities emerged from the Buffalo experiment who would have a profound effect on faculty development in the next several decades. In 1959 the Commonwealth Fund funded a study and evaluation of medical education at the University of Illinois College of Medicine and George Miller was invited to be director of the Office of Research in Medical Education (ORME), a post he held for seventeen years. The charge was the establishment of a permanent center with the staff to function as change agents, not merely as professional resources. Attention was focused on student learning rather than staff teaching. It was Miller's position that the most profound impact on the nature of learning was the examination system rather than the specification of objectives, the organization of the curriculum, or the quality of the instruction (Miller 1980).

The next organized institutional medical education unit was established in 1963 as the Division of Research in Medical Education (DRME) at the University of Southern California under the leaderhip of Stephen Abrahamson. Linkage with the School of Education was established in the beginning. Abrahamson was given academic appointments in both the School of Medicine and the School of Education. In addition he was invited to give a graduate seminar on education in the professions, and he offered research assistant opportunities in DRME to graduate students in education. By 1965 the USC Division of Research in Medical Education won national prominence with SIM I, a computerized trainer for anesthesiologists, and with the production of a single-concept film series on the neurologic examination and development of programmed patients as instructional aids. Some of the educational technology such as programmed patients has been widely exported into education and performance assessment. The focus on training tools was an impact directly felt by faculty at the institution. Howard Barrows, a colleague of Abrahamson, would soon move to McMaster to become involved in developing such teaching technologies as the standardized patient and triple jump assessment measures, which ultimately enhanced problem-based learning (Barrows and Tamblyn 1980).

By 1966 Hilliard Jason had moved on to the Michigan State University College of Human Medicine to establish the Office of Medical Education Research and Development (OMERAD), which was funded by the Commonwealth Fund. OMERAD was established as an independent unit and was represented on all educational policy committees. The formation of a new medical school curriculum by the collaboration of biomedical content experts and educational process experts was unique. The educational program "emphasized individualized learning and student responsibility for achieving defined professional competence, de-emphasized conventional grades and grading, highlighted the attitudinal goals of medical education and the interpersonal skills that are essential in the delivery of optimal health care, and fostered achievement of these goals by incorporating early clinical experience and giving equal emphasis to social/behavioral and bio-medical sciences" (Miller 1980). As well as creating a new educational program, OMERAD was charged with designing and implementing a longitudinal measure of student progress with respect to program objectives. Development of degree and nondegree programs in preparation for careers in medical education was also expected. For Jason, the process of learning was integral to education, and it was the philosophy of the unit to stress process over content and assessment. Jason was instrumental in establishing the NFME-funded seminal research on problem solving among physicians (Elstein et al. 1978). In addition, Jason's office was developed at the same time that Michigan State University College of Human Medicine (CHM) established its preclinical curriculum. The college of Human Medicine would be the early experimenter with problem-based learning in the United States.

DEVELOPMENT OF MEDICAL EDUCATION UNITS WITHIN SCHOOLS

Between 1959 and 1962 funding support became an important issue in the survival of research in medical education. While Miller at Illinois stressed that methods of student evaluation are more important than the quality of faculty teaching skills in promoting student learning, throughout the country the focus shifted to research improvement of faculty teaching rather than student learning. In 1960 the American Heart Association (AHA) initiated programs in continuing medical education organized by the University of Illinois ORME and established a grant-in-aid program that made it possible for medical schools to hold faculty retreats planned and conducted by established medical education research units. Two of the first schools to receive these grants, Hahnemann Medical College and Ohio State University, later went on to create their own medical education development and research programs. In 1961 the AHA established a fellowship program which sponsored a basic or clinical scientist to receive a year of training in an established department of research in medical education and to participate in the investigative programs thereof.

In 1952 the AAMC established national summer teaching institutes which occurred annually through 1961. These brought together medical educators, social and behavioral scientists, and professional educators. In 1962 the focus was shifted to a single school activity rather than a national meeting, and the first school to participate was the University of Kansas. The sponsor (AAMC) and the staff (consultants from the University of Illinois) learned that a seminar for forty faculty from a single school was very different from presenting comparable content to representatives of many schools. Adversarial rather than collegial relationships seemed to form, and hence substantial modification of format occurred in the programs offered in 1963–66. In an effort to promote institutional self-study by a local planning committee including faculty and administration who selected the parts of the local educational program to be studied, the new intramural seminars had shared leadership between the local committee and the educational consultants recruited by the AAMC. The University of Maryland, Tulane University, Ohio State University, and the Medical College of Georgia participated. The methods of study, the process of program organization and implementation, the content, and the outcome were described in Paul Sanazaro's report to the AAMC entitled "Educational Self-Study by Schools of Medicine."

The AAMC, under Ward Darley's leadership, established a Division of Education which was funded by a large grant from the Carnegie Corporation (Darley 1954). In 1962 the program was launched as a summer teaching institute. Within months after Hale Ham suggested that separate meetings be held at the annual AAMC meetings for those members doing research in medical education, a planning committee including Sanazaro, Ham, John Ginther, Milton Horowitz, Miller, George Reader, and Rosinski was formed and the meeting planned. Forty-one abstracts were received and sixteen papers were presented at the first annual Conference on Research in Medical Education in October 1962.

Also starting in 1962 was a medical education program at the Albany Medical College under the leadership of Frank Husted, one of Abrahamson's graduate students at Buffalo. A major contribution to medical education was Husted's seminar series on educational process for hospital residents. Because house officers carry a major responsibility for the teaching of medical students on the wards, the seminars' goal was to enhance the house officers' teaching skills. An additional benefit was the new insight provided on how to more effectively carry out such an introductory intervention for residents in the future (Miller 1980).

IMPACT OF MEDICAL EDUCATION ON FACULTY

By 1966 the "big three" medical education research and development programs (Illinois, Southern California, and Michigan State) had been established. By 1971, at the University of Illinois, thirty-five fellows completed one year of training, with most earning an M.Ed. degree and four a Ph.D. in education. Eventually some seventy-five fellows in medical education were graduated from the University of Southern California, Michigan State, Ohio State, and the University of Washington, although, unlike Illinois, most trainees were from the discipline of professional education. By 1977 seventy-two medical schools in the United States and Canada had clearly established units of educational research and development. Only five were officially recognized as academic departments. Formal graduate programs were being offered by nine units, and in all but one the college or school of education collaborated to provide an experience in health professions education.

In 1977, Jason's survey of faculty development determined the extent of impact of these units of medical education research and development on teaching in United States medical schools. It queried a random sample of 2,700 medical school faculty members from a total population of 27,393 about their preparation for teaching, their instructional practices in dealing with education problems, and their willingness to accept external assistance for finding solutions to these problems. The results revealed that only 21 percent had ever taken courses in education and only 39 percent had ever attended an educational workshop. Encouraging was the response that a large number of faculty were ready to accept help in improving their teaching skills. Although most preferred turning to their colleagues for help, many were ready to use specialists in educational process (Jason and Westberg 1982).

The university-affiliated faculty development movement which began in 1958 at the University of Buffalo gradually shifted focus. With the introduction of problem-based learning and interest in competency-based measurement, focus moved toward the process of teaching and problem solving itself. With the introduction of problem-based learning at McMaster University in 1969 and its experimentation at New Mexico, Michigan State University, and Rush, persons involved in the Buffalo experiment were also prime supporters of the problem-based movement. The recent interest in competency assessment has also emerged with defined implications for faculty development. The prevailing interest at the present time is on professional performance goals and health care outcomes (Miller 1980). The move to validate specialty board certification process and to identify the critical components of competence was initiated in 1964 by the American Board of Orthopaedic Surgeons in collaboration with the Illinois Office of Research in Medical Education and extended through 1972. This work paved the way for similar subsequent investigations in pediatric cardiology (with the USC group), in child psychiatry (with the Illinois group), and in emergency medicine (with the Michigan State group). The significance of the orthopaedic training study was that it was the beginning of support for medical education research from within individual practice specialties. Although not a faculty development project, it was the beginning of individual specialty associations picking up the banner of medical education.

COMPETENCY-BASED FACULTY DEVELOPMENT: FAMILY MEDICINE

In the 1970s family practice became recognized as an academic discipline and the number of family practice education programs grew rapidly. Because of its relatively brief history as an academic discipline and its lack of heritage possessed by the other academic medical disciplines, family practice chose to develop faculty as qualified teachers and academicians (Knopke and Anderson 1981). In an attempt to attract and prepare family physicians as faculty for the rapidly increasing number of residency programs (380 since 1969) and departments and divisions of family medicine (115 since 1969), faculty development fellowship programs have been established with financial support from the Division of Medicine of the U.S. Department of Health and Human Services, private foundations such as the Robert Wood Johnson Foundation and the Kellogg Foundation, and state governments (Hitchcock et al. 1980). When Bland et al. in 1987 studied the alumni of seventeen programs (1978–86) supported by the Robert Wood Johnson Foundation (RWJ) and the U.S. Department of Health and Human Services (HHS) there were 329 alumni in all, 262 from HHS programs and 67 from the RWJ programs. Of the 243 respondents, 140 held full-time faculty positions, 24 held paid part-time faculty positions, 35 were volunteer preceptors, and 44 had no teaching affiliation. All RWJ fellowships were for family practice physicians for two full years. There were 59 HHS programs studied that used a variety of educational formats, from day-long workshops to long-term fellowships (five weeks [62 per cent of the HHS alumni] to 12 months). The HHS fellowships were established to increase the number of full-time family physician faculty members and to improve the teaching skills of new and current faculty members, and the RWJ fellowships to prepare family physician faculty members in the skills needed to advance academic research in family medicine. The emphasis of the programs was on research skills, written communication skills, teaching skills, administration skills, and professional academic skills.

COMPETENCY-BASED FACULTY DEVELOPMENT: SOCIETY FOR GENERAL INTERNAL MEDICINE

General Internal Medicine divisions, in an attempt to establish their usefulness in academic research-oriented departments of internal medicine and to ensure their survival, have developed considerable interest in faculty development activities. The majority of general internal medicine faculty members studied by Linn et al. (1987) prefer learning in a small group taught by an expert. The Task Force on the Medical Interview of the Society of General Internal Medicine (SGIM) developed a series of faculty training workshops designed to teach faculty how to teach the interview. The task force originally was conceived out of a concern about the lack of adequate interviewing skills demonstrated by house staff. The purpose for integrating interviewing skills into graduate and postgraduate medical curricula was based on a belief in the importance of understanding psychosocial information in the development of the humanistic internist. Although initially structured to offer regional workshops to area faculty, the task force is also working within single institutions to meet articulated needs for faculty development. At the present time task force participants are working with the faculty at the University of New Mexico School of Medicine to offer faculty training workshops with the school's community preceptors who live and work throughout New Mexico. Task force participants are also working with faculty at Dartmouth Medical School to provide an integrated approach to teaching the medical interview.

In addition to the active participation of SGIM in faculty development, federal monies are now available to individual Departments of General Internal Medicine and General Pediatrics for creating programs for faculty development. A recently published federal report which reviews the past ten years of house staff training programs funded by the federal government recommended funding support for programs where all three primary care departments collaborated, developed, and provided faculty development programs.

Faculty development in the 1980s has assumed a different importance than when it began in the 1950s. Then it was critical to prove the need for such programs, and Miller, Jason, and Abrahamson set out to demonstrate the effectiveness of teaching faculty. In the 1980s the value of such programs is unquestioned. The vast technologic and information explosion has made the understanding of medical student learning critical for the effective and efficient relay of information in medical school. Now patients are more educated as well. They no longer accept the authority of the physician, and they often demand negotiating status in delivery of their own care. In addition, with the advances in medical research and treatment, the diseases seen in medical practice are more degenerative and chronic in nature than they were thirty-five years ago. Cancer was once considered a dramatic life-threatening disease. As a result of technological advances in oncology and hematology, many patients continue to live with the disease in much the same way someone might live with a chronic condition. The oncologist is now called upon to treat many patients with a view toward enhancing their coping and pain management skills and to work with them toward developing the highest quality of life possible.

Since the Buffalo experiment in the early 1950s, education has emerged as an important discipline. Faculty development has become the beacon of the movement in the last decade. With the introduction of problem-based learning and the emphasis on the process of teaching rather than the content, and with the concern among specialities for the discipline's integrity, has come a renewed interest in the purpose for which Buffalo started its experiment. Interestingly, the integral people involved at Buffalo can be traced to many educational innovations presently occurring in the United States and Canada. The seeds were sown for medical education to be responsive to many innovations and teaching technologies.

It would appear that the area of faculty development presently needs to have two frames of reference. The word *doctor* is derived from the Latin *docere*, to teach. Not only is student learning essential, but also patient learning. It is no surprise that the banner of faculty development is now being carried by the primary care specialities, family practice and general internal medicine, the practice groups most revered for their interpersonal skills and emphasis on the doctor/patient relationship. Although these practice groups have chosen to cement their place in the academic arena by establishing themselves as quality teachers of medical students and house staff, they are, in addition, those physicians as a group most qualified and most committed to patient education and patient learning.

Conclusions

Our goal in this chapter has been to describe a variety of innovative programs in order to draw some conclusions about humanism in medical education. Such a goal is no easy task. Innovative programs are occurring across the country in medical schools which vary in size, age of institution, mission, direction, and faculty desire. We believe, however, that the pattern of educational experimentation is toward small-group learning and away from the lecture method, toward the introduction of the patient early in the student's career, and toward bringing some form of ambulatory care experience into the clinical years. Many of these reforms have humanistic overtones. Any faculty member who has tutored in problem-based small groups has experienced a honeymoon relationship with his or her students which has often removed the traditional student/teacher boundaries from the learning interaction. Such an experience has provided the students with an opportunity to work more closely with the faculty and has set the stage for faculty to become excited by their work with the students. At the University of New Mexico, students in the traditional track were more apt to develop the "secret societies" found in Becker's work in medical education. These students demonstrated a strong network of informal groups where certain negative attitudes toward the faculty and the school were evident. Students in the experimental track (PCC) evidenced a far more comfortable relationhip with the faculty and did not seem to become involved in the strong informal groups evident in the traditional track and more easily portrayed a certain comfort with their training which was reminiscent of the socialization patterns found in the Cornell study. While medical students in the traditional track may have experienced similar socialization patterns toward the ultimate goal of becoming a physician (these medical students dealt with the difficulties of dissecting the cadaver as did the PCC students) the overriding concern among this group was with their discomfort with being in medical school. PCC students, on the other hand, seemed more at ease with the concept of their newly found professional identity. Neither group of students could be described as more "humanistic" in their later work with patients; yet the PCC students seemed generally "happy" to be in medical school.

Those programs which teach students to develop appropriate learning strategies have found that students perform better and describe the school as "warmer" and "more helpful" than they had expected medical school to be. Students introduced to patients early in their career also find a sense of purpose and relevance in their medical education not easily experienced in studying the basic sciences. They are able to move from an identification with the patient which dominates the first year of medical school and are able to appreciate the subtleties and ambiguity of clinical decision making before they are called upon to make decisions.

Although none of these programs is totally driven by the mission of humanism, does this diminish the impact which innovations might have on humanism? Probably not, and if the programs described above make any difference it may be in the direction of making medical education a more meaningful supportive environment for both students and faculty. What may be lacking in the programs reviewed above is a well-developed, longitudinal evaluation of the programs' effects on students' attitudes and values concerning medicine. Little research has appeared which would adequately document the impact which innovations have had on students' orientation to the medical profession.

Two surveys of outcomes research on innovations within medical education have been reported in the 1980s. Siu et al. (1987) examined all programs which had published evaluation results during the 1970s and early 1980s. His attempt was to describe what effect innovations have had on meeting the new challenge of preparing physicians for dealing with ethical dilemmas, modern technology, physician/patient relationships, increasing science base, and cost containment. Siu's conclusion was that "short term programs not integrated into the medical school environment are not worth pursuing. A more radical restructuring of medical education is needed." In addition, he felt that many of the newer innovations needed "to be more aggressively studied." Schmidt et al. (1987), in examining innovations currently occurring in problem-based and community oriented programs, found few differences between innovative schools and traditional programs in areas of performance outcomes. They also echoed others' results when they reported that community-oriented programs seem to have a higher rate of students entering primary care specialties. Such limited results are disappointing. This may be a result of the reliance on such traditional performance measures as NBME for comparative evaluation. Partly this is due to the inadequacy of appropriate measures which would describe the programs' impact on its students, and partly it is a result of the high quality of all medical students who will perform well regardless of the hurdles set in their path. More carefully documented studies which replicate the early study designs of Becker and Merton are needed to focus on the impact of educational innovations on developing and sustaining students' values toward humanistic medical practice.

Perhaps with the exception of the State University of New York at Buffalo and Western Reserve University, few innovative programs are old enough to have had an opportunity to follow their graduates into practice in order to examine the full impact of the program. Graduates of the Buffalo experiment are presently very active in medical education innovations and faculty training. The one undergraduate program, Western Reserve, has been in existence long enough to examine its graduate's career choices. Results from an evaluation conducted several decades after the Western Reserve experiment was in place found that there was a quantum leap of its graduates entering academic medicine which has been attributed to the curricular changes occurring in the 1950s.

Although innovations have been occurring over the past decades most are limited by certain structural parameters within medical education. These parameters have dominated the manner in which medical education is organized and may be the major stumbling block to any substantial reform. As we discussed earlier, this structure has its roots in an academic tradition which has successfully distinguished itself as a profession. However, like many other professions its emphasis on standardization of academic preparation has resulted in few major educational innovations. The manner in which medical education is organized is highly functional, yet within such a structure may lie the barriers to a more humanistic education. The major components of medical education are: (1) The Departmental structure of medical education where the objectives and required knowledge base is determined within each department or discipline. This results in large amounts of data to be memorized with few attempts to relate the relevance of the material to the future role of physician. (2) The lock step approach where students are taught the basic sciences within the first two years and the clinical sciences in the second two years with little connection between the two, either in content taught or in the style of teaching. (3) The reliance on the lecture method as the dominant mode of teaching, and content examination for assessing information retention during the first two years of medical school with a group of adult learners who have a variety of learning styles. (4) A faculty promotion policy which is based on research endeavors rather than teaching experience, leaving faculty with little interest in providing new and stimulating ways to communicate their fund of knowledge. (5) The reliance on house staff to provide the majority of teaching during the second two years of medical training with no formal preparation for teaching, except the dominant pedagogical model, "see one, do one, teach one." (6) The reliance on the tertiary care or university hospital–based setting to teach clinical medicine. Such a reliance assures consistency of information and up-to-date medical procedures and technology and reduces the lack of controlled standard which had previously existed in the pre-Flexnerian ambulatory care setting. It also places the control of teaching medicine within the hospital rather than the medical school domain.,

At the 1988 AAMC meetings two issues provided the challenge for the upcoming years in medical education. One concern rests with the very poor national performance on National Boards I. The second issue revolved around why the GPEP Report had not been implemented as had been originally intended. The two issues are symbolic of what confronts medical education at this juncture. The strength of NBME I has in numerous ways set parameters on innovations occurring in the United States. Their presence has forced innovative programs, in the final analysis, to produce students who will do as well on national boards as their colleagues from traditional programs. In many ways NBME is a product of the traditional lock step structure and represents the compartmentalization of learning which is a norm for medical education. The GPEP Report signaled a concern among educators about the process of teaching and learning in medical education. With its focus on improving the process of medical education, it was heralded as another Flexnerian revolution. There are yet no answers to the question of the two "failures," yet their mutual occurrence underlies the tension between the two. The scientific content has traditionally dominated the process of learning. With the increasing concern about how medicine is taught and its implications for humane and competent physicians, educators may take a more critical look at the values engendered by the present system of education. A revolution of sorts may be occurring. Such a revolution may not be defined by its political definition of "upheaval" but in its geometric one of revolving back to its beginning (Cohen 1985). We may have come full circle back to Flexner's original concern. Medical education has mastered the issue of standardization of competence and in so doing has strengthened the scientific basis of medicine. In that same process, the early emphasis on patient-oriented education may have been left behind.

Two incidents occurred—one at the University of New Mexico and the other at Dartmouth Medical School—which illustrate the concern abut the conservative force of the traditional mode upon the individual medical student. In 1981 at New Mexico, all students from the innovative problem-based curriculum were required to attend the traditional behavioral science lectures because the program directors believed not enough attention had been given to the psychosocial aspects of medicine in the tutorial groups. Students were expected to attend all of the lectures and small-group sessions. A response by one of the innovative track students characterized the group's reaction to attending the lectures: "I was so angry at myself. After a year of PCC to go to lectures and to regress to my old pattern of responding. I stopped reading for the class; I really just sat and waited for the lecturer to tell me what I needed to know." The student's description of what was obviously a contradiction of normative behavior in her learning pointed to an interesting issue. First, students confronted with lectures become passive and uninterested. Second, and perhaps more important, students, regardless of what preceded the experience, adapt to the next experience quite unconsciously, even if it may contradict what went before.

At Dartmouth Medical School, all students receive substantial information about alcoholism and addiction. The information is given around patients and is presented as part of the concern about student and physician impairment. Students receive this information in lectures in psychiatry and are expected to learn more about alcoholism on their psychiatric clerkship rotation. An evaluation of the effectiveness of the alcohol program indicated that students felt that they had a great deal of information about alcoholism, were comfortable dealing with alcoholism with patients, and would be comfortable dealing with colleagues if alcoholism arose as a problem. It seemed clear from student perceptions that they had learned a great deal about the nature of alcoholism and its importance in health care.

An interesting contradiction arose when students were videotaped in another clerkship setting. All primary care clerkship students are required to conduct an interview with a simulated patient. In spite of the training and the perceived expertise in treating alcoholism, almost no student inquired about alcoholism during the interview. Why do students who are in a school with extensive education in alcohol and addiction abuse, who expressed a sense of comfort in dealing with such content with a patient, not readily use this information in a simulated patient encounter? A further review of student responses in the evaluation questionnaire indicated that they reported little to no reinforcement in the clerkships other than primary care and psychiatry. Although they had learned the information, they had no support in applying it.

Medical education as it is presently structured appears to be a series of disparate events relying on the individual student to bridge the differences and to find the meaning in these varied experiences. In many ways students have to adapt to a certain structure of education which is forced upon them; survival and resulting competitiveness depends on how well they can accommodate. Sylvia Ashton-Warner (1936), who taught Maori children in New Zealand, wrote of the critical importance of recognizing cultural differences in education. Ashton-Warner believed that the teacher must find the students' "organic mode" of learning—their individual style of understanding the world. She related experiences in helping students combine their inner understanding with the outer world of education. If one can extend her message to professional school, it would seem that we are all subject to some form of cultural deprivation whenever we enter formal education. Anyone entering medical school enters a foreign environment with its own set of values and norms. Are we prepared to help students deal with their initial resistance to a new environment and also help these students learn this new information in as appropriate a manner as possible? This is a critical question in medical education when students are required to learn from such a variety of disciplines and from a faculty with differing and sometimes contradictory expectations.

We think quite easily of trying to find ways to stimulate a child's learning as effectively as possible but do not consider such an approach when educating adults. Medical schools have traditionally been arranged in a rigid manner of education and training, which continues into residency training. Within each step or stage of training are individual departments, disciplines, or specialities: biochemistry is taught by a biochemist, physiology by a physiologist. Internal medicine operates very differently from surgery, psychiatry from obstetrics/gynecology. Students move through each rotation, picking out the specialist's attitudes toward the patient, the individual physician's values toward technology, and their unique appreciation of psychosocial information in understanding the patient. What they learn to value in one specialty may not be highly valued in another. As a result, students seem to operate in a very case-specific manner, quickly learning that what they take from one area cannot be easily transported to another—or, as the teacher of the Maori would state, the information has been understood but not integrated.

The lack of integration starts early in the medical students' careers. What students have picked up in their first two years cannot be easily translated into their second two years. Often, what they learn about patients in one rotation may not be used in another rotation. If students learn the value of bioethics and psychosocial factors in psychiatry, will they readily transfer this information to an obstetrics/gynecology clerkship where such attitudes may not be so strongly supported? Such academic fragmentation is a product of medical education tradition, and few medical schools have attempted to integrate the basic sciences into the clinical sciences or provide a year of clerkship experience before teaching basic sciences. Schools such as Case Western Reserve and Harvard are attempting to provide students with longitudinal experiences which integrate learning the basic sciences with the clinical aspects of medicine. Case Western Reserve's organ system approach became the early method of teaching the relevance of the basic sciences and primarily remained within the first two years of medical education. Harvard is presently attempting to extend its new pathway concept throughout the second two years of clinical clerkships. The majority of innovations to date have occurred within the lock step structure limiting the integration of information. The implications for humanism in medical education are important. It may not be enough to teach a course on bioethics; students will learn the information but may not apply it in a clinical setting. It may not be enough to teach ambulatory care issues in a primary care clerkship, for students will probably not transfer such values as patient negotiation onto the wards. It is not enough to provide a "humanistic" environment for students in the first two years if in their clerkship years and residency training they suffer under unrealistic expectations and performance demands.

In this chapter we have described the histories of various programs which have attempted changes in learning environments. In addition, we have pointed to certain factors, mainly organizational, within medical education that continue to present major obstacles in the path of educational innovations. For the optimists among us, medical education would appear to have begun the process of reform, resulting in creative programs and exciting new educational technologies. For the more pessimistic of us, perhaps there is still much more to be considered and far more changes ahead. In the final analysis, the ultimate product—the competent, human-istic, scientist/physician—is a complex and elusive goal. As Flexner (1925) wrote:

> We have made it harder to achieve than need be by overloadng the curriculum. The remedy is to do less for the student rather than to do more. . . . But when the curriculum has been simplified, defects and disappointments will not disap-pear; these, due largely to human frailty, cannot be exorcised by jugglery. Far more wholesome would it be to admit once for all the *difficulty of learning* medicine and the *impossibility* of *teaching* it.

REFERENCES

AAMC (1984). *Physicians for the Twenty-First Century.* The GPEP Report. Association of American Medical Colleges, Washington, D.C.

Ashton-Warner, S. (1963/1986). *Teacher.* New York: Touchstone/Simon and Schuster.

Balint, M. (1972). *The Doctor, His Patient, and the Illness.* New York: International University Press.

Barrows, H. (1976). *Simulated Patients,* 2d ed. Springfield, Ill.: Charles C. Thomas.

Barrows, H., and Tamblyn, R. (1977). The portable patient problem pack: A problem based learning unit. *Journal of Medical Education,* 52, 1002–1004.

Barrows, H. and Tamblyn, R. (1980). *Problem-Based Learning: An Approach to Medical Education.* New York: Springer, p. 6.

Barzansky, B., Bussigel, G., Grenholm, G., and Richards, R. (1983). Planned curric-ulum change: A comparative case study. Presented at the annual meeting of the American Educational Research Association, Montreal.

Becker, H., Geer, B., Hughes, C., and Strauss, A. (1961). *Boys in White: Student Culture in Medical School.* Chicago: University of Chicago Press.

Bishop, C. (1988). Using male teaching associates to teach the genital-rectal exam. Innovations in Medical Education exhibit at the annual conference of the American Association of Medical Colleges.

Bland, C., Reineke, R. A., Welsh, W., and Shahady, E. (1979). Effectiveness of faculty development workshop in family medicine. *Journal of Family Practice,* 9, 453–458.

Bloom, S. (1973). *Power and Dissent in the Medical School.* New York: Free Press.

Brazeau, N., Jones, J., Hickner, J., and Vantassel, J. (1987). The Upper Peninsula medical education program and the problem based preclinical alternative. In *Innovative Tracks at Established Institutions for the Education of Health Personnel* M. Kantrowitz et al. (eds.). Geneva: World Health Organization.

Bridge, E. (1959). Experimental projects in medical teaching. *Journal of Medical Education,* 29, 17–24.

Camroe, J. (1953). The achievements of the institute: Report of the first teaching institute. American Association of Medical Colleges, Atlantic City, *Journal of Medical Education,* 98–162.

Cohen, J. B. (1985). *Revolution in Science.* Cambridge, Mass.: Harvard University Press.

Colby, K., Almy, T., and Zubkoff, M. (1986). Problem-based learning of social sciences and humanities by fourth year students. *Journal of Medical Education*, 61, 413–415.

Coombs, R. H., and Boyle, B. P. (1971). The transition to medical school: Expectations versus realities. In *Psychosocial Aspects of Medical Training*, Coombs and C. H. Vincent (eds.). Springfield, Ill.: Charles C. Thomas.

Darly, W. (1954). Medical education and the potential of the student to learn. *Journal of Medical Education*, 11–20.

Dietrich, A., Garrett, E., and Caldwell, J. (1986). Medical student teaching in the preclinical years: A national family medicine survey. *Family Medicine*, 18, 3, 136–139.

Durinzi, D. (1988). Application of a clinical skills evaluation data base: Design, development, findings, and future use. Innovations in Medical Education exhibit at the annual conference of the American Association of Medical Colleges.

Elstein, A., Schulman, L., and Spratfka, S. (1978). *Medical Problem Solving: An Analysis of Clinical Reasoning*. Cambridge, Mass.: Harvard University Press.

Eminson, M. (1988). Teaching medical students new approaches to communicating the diagnosis of handicap. Innovations in Medical Education exhibit at the annual conference of the American Association of Medical Colleges.

Farber, M., and Altman, L. (1988). A great hospital in crisis. *New York Times Magazine*, January 24, 18–21.

Farquhar, L. (1988). Investigating the relationship between knowledge and attitudes: AIDS and the medical student. Innovations in Medical Education exhibit at the annual conference of the American Association of Medical Colleges.

Flexner, A. (1925). *Medical Education: A Comparative Study*, New York: Macmillan.

Fox, R. (1989). *The Sociology of Medicine: A Participant Observer's View*. Englewood Cliffs, N.J.: Prentice-Hall.

Friedman, C. (1988). Inquirer: A database for microbiology. Innovations in Medical Education exhibit at the annual conference of the American Association of Medical Colleges.

Funkenstein, D. H. (1968). The learning and personal development of medical students and the recent changes in universities and medical schools. *Journal of Medical Education*, 43, 883-897.

Gelula, M. and Moore, M. (1988). Skills for lifelong learning. Innovations in Medical Education exhibit at the annual conference of the American Association of Medical Colleges.

Gordon, G., and Rost, K. (unpublished). Evaluating the SIGM task force faculty development course on teaching the medical interview.

Gotterer, G., Blumbert, P., and Paul, H. (1987). The alternative preclinical curriculum. In *Innovative Tracks at Established Institutions for the Education of Health Personnel*. M. Kantrowitz, et al. (eds.). Geneva: World Health Organization.

Harris, D., Coleman, M., and Mallea, M. (1982). Impact of participation in a family practice track program on student career decision. *Journal of Medical Education*, 57, 609–614.

Harris, D., and Effert, P. (1983). Effects of clinical preceptorship on career and practice site choices. *West Journal of Medicine*. 138, 2, 276–279.

Hess, G. (1988). An authoring system for computer-based patient management simulations. Innovations in Medical Education exhibit at the annual conference of the American Association of Medical Colleges.

Hitchcock, M. A., Ramsey, C. W., and Herring, M. (1980). A model for developing clinical teaching skills of family practice teachers. *Journal of Family Practice*, 11, 923–929.

Jason, H. (1987). Foreword, *Implementing Problem-Based Medical Education: Lessons from Successful Innovations*. Arthur Kaufman (ed.). New York: Springer.

Jason, H., and Westberg, J. (1982). *Teachers and Teaching in U.S. Medical Schools,* Norwalk, Conn.: Appleton-Century-Crofts.

Jonas, S. (1978). *Medical Mystery: The Training of Doctors in the United States.* New York: Norton.

Kantrowitz, M., Kaufman, A., Mennin, S., Fulop, T., and Guilbert, J. (eds.) (1987). *Innovative Tracks at Established Institutions for the Education of Health Personnel.* Geneva: World Health Organization, Offset Publication No. 101.

Kantrowitz, M., and Kaufman, A. (1985). International perspectives. In *Implementing Problem-Based Medical Education: Lessons from Successful Innovations.* Arthur Kaufman (ed.). New York: Springer.

Kaufman, A. (ed.) (1985). *Implementing Problem-Based Medical Education: Lessons from successful innovations.* New York: Springer.

Kaufman, A. (1988). The New Mexico experiment: From problem based learning to social medicine. *GME Correspondent,* 1.

Kennell, J., Chickering, D., and Soroker, E. (1961). Experience with a Medical School Family Study. *Journal of Medical Education,* 36, 1649–1716.

Knopke, H. J., and Anderson, R. L. (1981). Academic development in family practice. *Journal of Family Practice,* 12, 493–499.

Knowles, M., (1970). *The Modern Practice of Adult Education: Andragogy versus Pedagogy.* New York: Association Press.

Leiden, L. (1988). Learning styles: Implications for students and faculty. GME presentation at the annual conference of the American Association of Medical Colleges.

Linn, L.S., Lewis, C.E., and Leake, B.D. (1987). Faculty development in general internal medicine: Perception concerning academic survival. *Archives of Internal Medicine,* 147, 1446–1451.

Lloyd, C., and Gartrell, J.K. (1983). A further assessment of medical school stress. *Journal of Medical Education,* 58, 984–967.

McDaniel, J. (1988). The development and design of a computerized call structure for a pediatric residency program. Innovations in Medical Education exhibit at the annual conference of the American Association of Medical Colleges.

Merton, R., Reader, C., and Kendall, P. (1957). *The Student Physician: Introductory Studies in the Sociology of Medical Education.* Cambridge, Mass.: Harvard University Press.

Mennin, S., Woodside, E., Bernstein, M., Kantrowitz, M., and Kaufman, A. (1987). Primary care curriculum. In *Innovative Tracks at Established Institutions for the Education of Health Personnel.* M. Kantrowitz, et al. (eds.). Geneva: World Health Organization.

Miller, G. (1980). *Training Medical Educators.* Cambridge, Mass.: Harvard University Press.

Mizrahi, T. (1986). *Getting Rid of Patients.* New Brunswick, N.J.: Rutgers University Press.

Moore-West, M., and O'Donnell, M. (1985). Program evaluation. In *Implementing Problem-Based Medical Education: Lessons from Successful Innovations.* Arthur Kaufman (ed.). New York: Springer.

Moore-West, M., Harrington, D., Mennin, S., and Kaufman, A. (1986). Distress and attitudes toward the learning environment: Effects of a curriculum innovation. *Proceedings of the Annual Conference on Research in Medical Education,* 25, 293–300.

Morantz-Sanchez, R. M. (1985). *Sympathy and Science: Women Physicians in American Medicine.* New York: Oxford University Press.

Myers, I. (1962). *The Myers-Briggs Type Indicator Manual.* Princeton, N.J.: Educational Testing Service.

Nelson, J., and Palmer, J. (1988). Introduction to medical school: An holistic approach to orientation. Presentation at the annual conference of the American Association of Medical Colleges.

Nutting, P. (ed.) (1987). Community-oriented primary care: From principle to practice. U.S. Department of Health and Human Services, Washington, D.C., HRSA Pub. No. HRS-A-PE-61.

O'Donnell, J. (1987). Personal communication concerning oncology/hematology survey; at the Association of Cancer Education, New Orleans.

Paterson, G. (1988). Student data from admissions to manpower planning. Innovations in Medical Education exhibit at the annual conference of the American Association of Medical Colleges.

Ramos, M., and Moore, G. (1987). The new pathway to medical education. In *Innovative Tracks at Established Institutions for the Education of Health Personnel.* M. Kantrowitz, et al. (eds.). Geneva: World Health Organization.

Robertson, C. A. (1960). A place of social medicine in medicine and in the medical curriculum. *Canadian Medical Association Journal*, 82, 724–726.

Robertson, C. A. (1960). Teaching comprehensive medical care. *Canadian Medical Association Journal*, 82, 734–735.

Schmidt, H., Dauphinee, W., and Patel, V. (1987). Comparing the effects of problem-based and conventional curricula in an international sample. *Journal of Medical Education*, 62, 305–315.

Shain, D. F., and Kelliher, G. (1988). A study skills workshop as an integral part of orientation to medical school: The establishment of self directed learning. Presentation at the annual conference of the American Association of Medical Colleges.

Siu, A., Mayer-Oakes, A., and Brook, R. (1987). Innovations in medical curricula: Templates in change? *Health Affairs*, 60–71.

Starr, P. (1982). *The Social Transformation of American Medicine.* New York: Basic Books.

Thornborough, J. (1988). The Mount Sinai School of Medicine self-testing system version 2. Innovations in Medical Education exhibit at the annual conference of the American Association of Medical Colleges.

Van Susteren, T. (1988). Attitude of medical professionals toward elderly patients: Development of a scale to measure change. Innovations in Medical Education exhibit at the annual conference of the American Association of Medical Colleges.

Voorhees, D., Bennett, M., Counsellor, A. (1985). Extended community preceptorship: Problem-based learning in the field. In *Implementing Problem-Based Medical Education: Lessons from Successful Innovations.* Arthur Kaufman (ed.). New York: Springer.

Willey, M. (1988). Utilization of peer-tutoring in a new academic development program. Innovations in Medical Education exhibit at the annual conference of the American Association of Medical Colleges.

Williams, G. (1980). *Western Reserve's Experiment in Medical Education and Its Outcome.* New York: Oxford University Press.

Willoughby, L. (1988). The challenge exam: Testing knowledge in specific content areas. Innovations in Medical Education exhibit at the annual conference of the American Association of Medical Colleges.

Woodbury, G., Harden, M., and Mullen, P. (1988). Evaluation of a structured personal development program for premedical minority students. Presentation at the annual conference of the American Association of Medical Colleges.

Zoccolillo, M. (1988). Major depression during medical training. Editorial in *JAMA*, 260, 2560-2561.

Wofford, D. (1987). Bowman Gray tries experimental method. *Tower Journal*, Winston-Salem, N.C., November 8.

TEN

Promoting the Adaptation and Coping of Pediatric Residents

MORRIS GREEN

An important role of the pediatrician is to help parents and children successfully adapt to and cope with the changing circumstances of their lives. Positive parental outcomes include self-confidence, self-esteem, and autonomy; enjoyment of parenthood; adequate family communication; maintenance of social supports; understanding of child development; nurturant parent-child interactions; a good marital relationship; and comfort in seeking help for current problems and major stressors. Maladaptive parental behaviors include inadequate parent-child interaction, child abuse, excessive use of health services, and under- or overstimulation of the child. Positive adaptive outcomes in children include the ability to communicate well, express fellings, relate positively to others, and develop trusting relationships. Other strengths of children are physical fitness, personal achievement, a constructive assessment of personal capacities, good grooming, self-responsibility for health, high self-esteem, and the security of being cared for and loved.

The promotion of adaptation is a long-established pediatric tradition (Green 1986). It has been the pediatrician's job to enhance a child's capacity to adapt to a variety of biologic stressors. The administration of antibiotics to an infant with bacteremia helps the baby successfully cope with and overcome a possibly fatal stressor. Measles immunization offers a prospective adaptation to the measles virus, a potentially deleterious biologic insult. Insulin contributes to a child's immediate metabolic adaptation to the physiologic derangements caused by juvenile diabetes.

Pediatric practitioners have the opportunity to facilitate mastery of those expected and unexpected transitions, events, and crises that test the coping repertoires of parents and children. As part of their day-to-day care, they have the opportunity to help children and their parents identify their strengths and resources, to suggest protective strategies, to intervene early, and to treat symptoms or problems that result from maladaptation.

Adaptation to changes and stresses may be (1) prospective, e.g., preparation for an adoption, for hospitalization, for surgery, for puberty or for the remarriage of a parent; (2) concurrent, e.g., coping with an infant with a difficult temperament, the birth of a baby with a handicap, parental separation, divorce, death, unemployment, suicide, homicide, accidents, sexual assault, serious illness, or the mother going to work outside the home; or (3) rehabilitative, e.g., providing care for the disorders and symptoms that result from maladaptation.

Stress has attracted much public and professional interest in recent years. Still relatively unexplored, however, is the adaptation and coping of medical students and physicians to the stressors that they confront in their daily lives. This area, in which the late Nancy Roeske had a special interest, will be the subject of this chapter.

The Adaptation of Pediatric Residents

Resident adaptation programs can, of course, be justified on humanitarian and ethical grounds alone, but at the same time they can serve to enhance patient care, contribute to pediatric education, and have a heuristic value for research. As pediatric services increasingly become centers for the care of seriously and critically ill children, the capacity of these services to provide adequate emotional support for their patients and their families may be importantly enhanced by acknowledging and addressing house staff stressors. In addition to their contributions to patient care, resident adaptation programs may also be of educational value in raising the level of consciousness of house officers to those life and developmental stressors commonly experienced by the patients and families (McCue 1982).

Pediatric House Staff Stressors

What are the stressors commonly encountered by pediatric residents (McCue 1985; Schaff and Hoekelman 1981; Butterfield 1988)? What are the consequences of such stresses? What are the protective or modifying factors that may buffer stress?

Table 1 lists episodic professional stressors for pediatric house staff. Encountered singly, individual stressors have one level of effect, some more than others, but when they occur in clusters or against a background of chronic or cumulative professional stresses such as those listed in table 2, their impact is greatly enhanced.

In addition to programmatic and professional stresses, individual residents are commonly confronted with one or more personal stressors such as those listed in table 3. While some are additive, others are multiplicative. Some are also more aversive than others. Residents who are experiencing several personal and professional stressors simultaneously are highly vulnerable (Small 1981).

Life as a physician is neither possible nor desirable without stress. Indeed, in measured amounts, stress seems to have a growth-promoting and steeling rather than merely a noxious effect. Positive outcomes that follow the exposure of residents to the kind of progressively more difficult challenges that they can reasonably master include the feelings of accomplishment and high self-esteem that are essential to a physician's optimal functioning. For example, learning how to deal with such recurrent professional stressors as the death of a child or how to adapt to experiences of failure leads not only to improved future performance in similar situations but also to enhanced personal and professional growth and a larger coping repertoire.

The physician's increased understanding of stressors, their consequences, and the contribution of protective and modifying factors may promote his or her empathy for patients who themselves are enduring

Table 1. Episodic Professional Stressors

Caring for critically ill patients and their parents.
Caring for dying patients and their parents.
Caring for an intensely anxious patient and/or family.
Lack of back-up by senior resident or attending physician when overwhelmed with work or lack of information.
Disagreement (usually nonverbalized) with attending physician about appropriateness of continued biomedical treatment of a dying child, especially if such treatment appears futile.
Incongruity between the needs of a child as perceived by the resident, parents, and attending physician.
Hostile, challenging, demanding, or threatening parents.
Being blamed by the parents directly or by implication for a child's death.
Parents who will not permit the resident to "touch" the patient.
Making a serious diagnostic or therapeutic mistake that causes death or handicap.
Being unfairly or publicly criticized by an attending physician.
Inability to relieve a patient's pain.
Inability to draw blood or start an intravenous line.
Caring for children who become physically deformed because of their illness.
Caring for a patient who is self-destructive.
Parents who seek to dictate and control the work-up and treatment.
Comatose patients or children who cannot respond socially.
Chronically ill patients who do not demonstrate improvement.
Dealing with physical or sexual abuse.
Multiproblem patients and families.
Conflict between time for work, for self, and for family.
Guilt about feeling relieved when a fatally ill patient dies.
Prescribing treatment that makes a child distressingly ill.
Involvement in unsuccessful resuscitation effort.

Table 2. Chronic or Cumulative Stressors

Inappropriately heavy workload or excessive responsibilities.

Sleep deprivation, physical fatigue.

Emotional fatigue, e.g., caring for an extended period for many dying or potentially dying patients.

Unremitting time pressures.

Insufficient training, information, and supervision in some areas.

Daily hassles, e.g., commuting, parking, personally difficult professional colleagues, bureaucracy, housing, inadequate day-care availability, excessive paging, or feeling of being just a cog in a large impersonal machine.

Feeling of being trapped in a set of circumstances that one cannot change; a sense of nonparticipation in the direction of the program.

Feeling of being on the outside looking in.

Incongruity between needs of a child as seen by the resident, the parents, and the attending physician.

Absence of appropriate praise or feedback regarding performance.

Monotonous, nonchallenging, and unduly repetitious duties.

No time to read.

Noncompliance or lack of expressed gratitude on the part of some parents.

Inadequate opportunities for physical activity, exercise, sports, dating, relaxation, and cultural activities.

Clustering of episodic professional stressors.

stresses. Similarly, such knowledge may augment the physician's ability to provide truly personal care of patients and promote the personal freedom that permits the physician to become an effective advocate for children and families. These experiences also encourage the emergence of those characteristics of master pediatric clinicians that are listed in table 4.

On the other hand, when an excessive number of personal or professional stressors are complemented by an insufficient number of protective or mediating factors, the coping capacities of the resident may be exceeded. At that point, symptoms may appear, e.g., irritability, contentiousness, suspiciousness, temper outbursts, and hostility to a family. Depressive symptoms may include insomnia, anorexia, overeating, lack of motivation, depressed mood, and withdrawal. Anxiety may account for uneven performance, indecisiveness, diagnostic and therapeutic errors, and overattachment to a family. With more severe degrees of maladaptation, there may be an increase in illness among the residents, marital difficulties, substance abuse, change in career plans, and suicide.

When behaviors and symptoms such as these surface in a residency program, prompt intervention is indicated, including assessment of the level of the stress in the program, discussions with the residents and faculty, and the rapid introduction of corrective measures.

The extent to which the adaptation of the residents is positive or negative can be heavily influenced by personal and group protective and modifying factors. The former include both those that are professionally related and those of a more widely applicable nature. The former include biomedical and psychosocial competence, the recognition and acceptance of the boundaries of one's current competency, a belief that one's work is meaningful, a sense of accomplishment, pride in one's daily performance, and the sense of belonging to a valued group.

Closely allied strengths include the ability to develop working alliances and positive relationships at work, the avoidance of situations in which one has no constructive role, the ability to withstand time pressures and to use time effectively, the capacity to identify professional stressors, the acceptance that such stressors are the inevitable accompaniment of the privilege of being a physician, and the recognition that physicians as well as patients have emotional needs.

Other personal attributes that contribute to a resident's resilience in the face of stress include an internal locus of control, the ability to define and persist in achieving goals, success in the mobilization of social supports, availability of friends and confidants, willingness to turn to others in times of stress, and comfort in asking for help. Additional attributes highly useful both within and outside the resident's workplace include the ability to be assertive in a constructive fashion, conflict resolution skills, a reasonably high threshold for the perception of experiences as stressful, mastery of previous stressful situations, high self-esteem, and the ability to attend to personal and family needs.

A house staff retreat early in the academic year provides an opportunity to prepare the residents prospectively for commonly encountered stressors. Such group anticipatory guidance helps the residents know what to expect and how to cope with selected stressful situations. Another group

Table 3. Personal Stressors

Death of a significant person.
Loneliness and isolation; inability to make friends; if single, lack of male or female friends.
Lack of social supports or a social network that is draining rather than supportive.
Role conflicts between being a resident, a spouse, and a parent.
Separation and divorce.
Marital problems.
Breakup of a close relationship.
Illness, including migraine headaches, arthritis, asthma.
Lack of time for personal activities.
Lack of gratification from work.
Unrealistically high self-expectations.
Anxiety, depression, substance abuse.
Hesitancy to ask questions.
Having a handicapped child.
Financial concerns.
Unanticipated change in night call or rotation schedule.

Table 4. Ten Characteristics of a Master Clinician

1. Highly secure about one's own medical competency.
2. Interested in persons and personal care as well as disease.
3. Able to *care* for others, especially those who experience adversity; projects personal warmth and empathy without being personally engulfed.
4. Recognizes, understands, and is reasonably comfortable in dealing appropriately with patients' feelings.
5. Aware of one's own feelings and reactions.
6. Has strategies to cope with personal discomfort.
7. Gracious, courteous, mature, and responsive.
8. Has well-developed professional linkages and secure personal support systems.
9. Able to deal with uncertainty.
10. Believes one's own personal and professional life is highly meaningful.

protective or stress-modifying factor has been termed the *human aggregate characteristics* of the environment—the general supportiveness, friendliness, courtesy, and helpfulness of the hospital staff and faculty that convey their investment in the education and well-being of the house staff.

Other useful group arrangements include carefully selected faculty advisers who meet with their advisees at least monthly for feedback and reassurance of worth, immediate opportunities for debriefing after a particularly stressful experience, early identification of residents who need help, and confidential access to marriage or personal counseling. It is important that the program director be alert to house staff applicants who may be at special risk, who may augment group vulnerability, or who may, on the other hand, contribute to group resiliency.

Supportive adminstrative arrangements within a residency program include changes of pace in the schedule, shared time opportunities, ready availability of day care, parental leaves, opportunity for personal days, spouse support groups, house staff discussion groups to identify problems and feelings, and social activities such as parties, dinners, picnics, skits, and sports.

Developing a Resident Adaptation Program

How does one develop a resident adaptation program for an individual residency (Berg and Garrard 1980; Siegel and Donnelly 1978)? One approach is through house staff–faculty problem-solving sessions in which content such as that included in the tables above is identified and discussed. Unstructured support sessions of faculty, house staff, and nurses are also useful, particularly in newborn and pediatric intensive care units, but their long-term effects are generally limited because they are not convened to develop solutions destined to be integrated into the program.

More structured sessions are advisable to identify and recommend which programmatic protective strategies to introduce, continue, or strengthen. Group cohesiveness and a working alliance develop when much of this work is done by the group as a whole with defined projects undertaken by subgroups of residents and faculty members.

Resident participation is essential, not only because residents have many constructive ideas to contribute but also because their joint authorship of changes helps ensure their implementation. Their meaningful participation in problem-solving also provides practical experience in how to be effectively assertive and constructive on behalf of themselves, their patients, their program, and their institution. Since two or three house staff representatives cannot truly portray the feelings and views of each resident, even though they attempt to do so in a balanced fashion, general participation is important. The process can be initiated with a retreat, if that can be easily arranged, but it needs to be continued during the year with a frequency of once a month or so.

Prospective or anticipatory house staff adaptation is a protective technique that warrants exploration. The notion that persons who are prepared for a stressful experience cope better than those who have not seems reasonable. Indeed, that is the justification for much of pediatric health supervision. Certainly pediatric residents can be prospectively prepared for a number of major stressors, e.g., dealing with a very hostile parent, making a diagnostic or therapeutic mistake, feeling overwhelmed, experiencing significant depression, or caring for a dying child.

A resident's ability to care for dying children and their parents depends heavily on conscious and unconscious personal reactions, personality structure, family experiences, and styles of coping. It would seem to be a reasonable hypothesis that the capacity of pediatric residents for their role in death, bereavement, and other stressful situations could be enhanced through the kind of education and preparation that equips them prospectively with the necessary knowledge base and clinical skills. As an example, house officers who have had an opportunity to explore their own feelings regarding death prior to having the professional opportunity to help children and parents confront it may be more likely to provide effective and compassionate care.

It would seem educationally useful to prepare anticipatory packages or protocols for several major resident stressors. Such educational modules could discuss the nature of the stressor, its effects, and methods of coping and adaptation. Such anticipatory guidance could enhance the residents' personal comfort; help with their personal anxiety, depression, grief, anger, guilt, and frustration; and facilitate their provision of effective and compassionate care.

REFERENCES

Berg JK, Garrard J: Psychosocial support in residency training programs. *J Med Educ* 1980;55:851.

Butterfield PS: The stress of residency: A review of the literature. *Arch Intern Med* 1988;148:1428.

Green M: Pediatric education and the care of the person. *Pediatrics* 1986;78:431.

McCue JD: The effects of stress on physicians and their medical practice. *N Engl J Med* 1982;306:458.

McCue JD: The distress of internship. *N Engl J Med* 1985;312:449.

Schaff EA, Hoekelman RA: Stressed interns. *Pediatrics* 1981;68:605.

Siegel B, Donnelly JC: Enriching personal and professional development: The experience of a support group for interns. *J Med Educ* 1978;55:908.

Small GW: House officer stress syndrome. *Psychosomatics* 1981;22:860.

ELEVEN

Reducing Stress in Medical Oncology House Officers

A Preliminary Report of a Prospective Intervention Study

KATHRYN M. KASH AND JIMMIE C. HOLLAND

Over the past ten years, much has been written about stress on interns and residents, but far fewer studies have tested interventions to alter the negative effects on their psychological and physical health. During that time, the stresses have only escalated as house officers have had to utilize more technical procedures and information in their patient care (McCue 1982). These stresses, related to medicine in general, are magnified even further in the modern cancer center where the house officer deals with diseases for which curative treatments are often limited and progressive disease and death are frequent outcomes.

This chapter focuses on an experimental intervention introduced to reduce stress on staff working on a medical oncology unit. It was our hypothesis that this intervention would also enable the staff to give more sensitive and compassionate care and consequently would have a positive effect on the patients' perceptions about the human aspects of their care. The controlled trial used a social systems intervention that was evaluated for its effectiveness in (1) ameliorating the deleterious effects of stress on the house staff and (2) improving patients' perception of their care. To place the study in perspective, a brief review of the stresses on house staff and some of the consequences is presented.

Stressors for Medical Students and House Officers

Men and women who enter medical schools bring with them certain personality characteristics that contribute to stress. Foremost are the strong obsessive-compulsive traits that led them to choose a career requiring long hours of study, heavy responsibility, and devotion to work. In fact, the more these traits are exaggerated, ironically, the more successful a student may be in his or her work (Reuben 1983). These traits, in conjunction with overly controlled emotions and low need for relaxation and pleasure, may render the medical student and house officer more vulnerable than others to depression, alcoholism, psychiatric disorders, and suicide. Medical students are also stressed by financial burdens, an overload of knowledge to be acquired, frequent challenges to their competence (especially in the clinical years), social isolation, fatigue, and the psychological discomfort of dealing with cadavers and later with dying patients for the first time (Gaensbauer and Mizner 1980).

While some of the above stressors are considered healthy, some have negative effects on both satisfaction and performance. For the house officer, loneliness, work overload, and new responsibilities for the care of seriously ill patients are major stresses. Interns and residents work eighty hours a week, often with on-call periods of thirty to thirty-six hours without sleep. Sleep loss and fatigue actually impair one's ability to think clearly and to assess information, as in reading electrocardiograms (Friedman et al. 1973). It is not surprising that a house officer stress syndrome described by Small (1981) includes episodic cognitive impairment due to lack of sleep, chronic anger and resentment about demands on time and energy, family discord (especially marital problems), and a pervasive cynicism. A more detailed review of the stresses on doctors in general medicine may be found elsewhere (Cartwright 1979).

The modern cancer center places novel stresses on both staff and patients as technology imposes more complex diagnostic procedures, monitoring devices, and treatments (e.g., Bard 1984; Holland 1982). Not only the technical side but also the emotional burdens of caring for patients who are extremely ill contribute to stresses (Vachon 1987). The frequent deaths of patients of all ages, staff conflicts and poor communications, intense involvement with patients and their families, and conflicts between research and clinical care goals make handling the workload difficult.

Both the gravity of the illness under treatment and the emphasis on clinical investigation make the modern cancer treatment setting quite similar to that of the metabolic research ward so elegantly described by Fox (1962). It was in such a research unit setting, over two decades ago, that the initial trials of steroids for previously fatal diseases were conducted. The same psychological problems appear today: dealing with uncertainty, frustration with failure, and concerns about outcome of often hopeless illness. Black humor, alliances with patients, and similar ways of coping are also seen. House officers are confronted with these problems and reactions when they rotate to an oncology unit or cancer center.

Consequences of Stress

During their education, one-third of medical students seek professional counseling because they suffer anxiety or depression secondary to academic pressures or because they feel emotional distance from others (Weinstein 1983). This is likely an underestimate of the number who actually need help, because many schools have inadequate counseling resources and some students fear the stigma and potential retaliation for seeking a psychiatric consultation. That suicide is the second leading cause of death among medical students speaks for the need for counseling and greater attention (Ross 1971).

As for house officers, one-third of the interns in one study reported significant depression during their internships; approximately 25 per cent stated they had had suicidal ideation (Valko and Clayton 1975). During the years 1979 to 1984, 55.5 percent of the internal medicine training programs granted leaves of absence to residents because of emotional problems (Smith et al. 1986). While 79 percent of these residents ultimately returned, 10 percent dropped out of medicine and 2 per cent committed suicide. A survey of 1805 interns, residents, and fellows in Ontario, Canada (Hsu and Marshall 1987), revealed that 23 percent had some degree of distress or depression on the Center for Epidemiological Studies of Depression Scale (CES-D). Among the men (N = 1162), interns had the highest frequency of depression and distress ranging from mild to severe, and 26 percent of them had high scores on the CES-D. Among the women (N = 585), interns again received the highest scores in the distress and depression ranges; 38 percent of these women had high scores on the CES-D.

Many physical stress-related symptoms are reported by house officers; these include tension headaches, gastrointestinal disturbances, exhaustion, fatigue, and insomnia. The "medical student syndrome" of hypochondriacal concerns is seen in all trainees working with cancer patients for the first time. A minor symptom, usually disregarded in other contexts, is seen as an early symptom of cancer, in oneself or a relative. Attempts at self-medication, along with frequent delay in seeking a consultation for a symptom, are common.

Coupled with such physical symptoms are signs of psychological distress: loss of enthusiasm for work, depression, irritability and frustration, and a cynical view of medicine and colleagues (Hall et al. 1979; Holland and Holland 1985; Maslach 1979; Mount 1986). The house officer shows excessive dedication and commitment, working longer hours but with less productivity and decreased sensitivity to the emotional needs of patients and others. Conversely, he or she may become detached and disinterested in medical practice.

These signs in health care professionals, described by Maslach (1979) as the "burnout" syndrome, apply to house staff. Emotional exhaustion, depersonalization, and lack of a sense of personal accomplishment are common. Emotional exhaustion is described as feeling emotionally overextended and exhausted by work. Depersonalization is a poor term, but it describes the sense of distance and reduced sympathy toward patients. Lack of personal accomplishment is felt: "What do I ever accomplish anyway?" In oncology, it is translated into the feeling that all cancer treatment is futile, so why bother. Another concept of burnout symptoms was proposed as a form of survivor syndrome in health caregivers who deal repeatedly with losses from death (Millerd 1977). Some of the adverse symptoms are the same as those seen in survivors of natural disasters.

Both the stressors and the consequences of stress outlined above led us to the conclusion that sufficient data exist on work-related stress. The research needed was a prospective trial of an intervention which, if shown to be effective, could be introduced in cancer units. Before we began we did a review of intervention strategies that have been reported as effective.

Intervention Strategies for House Officers

Consultation liaison psychiatry has most extensively studied patients' psychological reactions to illness and physicians' responses to giving clinical care (Strain and Hammerman 1978). The care of patients with life-threatening and fatal illnesses has long been identified as the most stressful kind of care, and those giving these services are in most need of psychological support (Spikes and Holland 1975). For oncology fellows the overall ideal support likely comes from having a single individual, usually a liaison psychiatrist, who constitutes a "psychological presence" in both inpatient and outpatient settings, and to whom problems can be brought without fear of ridicule or embarrassment (Artiss and Levine 1973).

Most efforts directed toward house staff distress have aimed at providing both group and individual assistance. Support groups were effective with pediatric house staff in promoting cooperation and reducing isolation (Siegel and Donnelly 1978). Special mental health programs, such as a free service at UCLA for psychiatric consultation and brief psychotherapy, have been effective (Borenstein and Cook 1982). Also, orienting new house staff, especially chief residents, to the psychological problems that may be anticipated among house staff more likely will assure their identification.

Rotations through oncology are often dreaded by medical residents, and most are ill-prepared for the complex care required or the large number of seriously ill and dying patients. Personal problems are often taken to the liaison psychiatrist as a known and trusted colleague. When this visibility on a medical oncology unit is coupled with close coordination with the chief resident, potential problems are identified and often averted.

At several institutions, interdisciplinary and single discipline group seminars or rounds on oncology units have been held to provide support (Artiss and Levine 1973; Richards and Schmale 1974; Wise 1977; Strain and Hammerman 1978). Although the formats and frequency of meetings vary, goals are similar. The main themes, focusing on the emotional needs and problems of the patients, help staff members cope with their feelings. At Memorial Sloan-Kettering Cancer Center (MSKCC), a weekly meeting has been held for the past five years on the neurooncology unit where dealing with patients with brain tumors is particularly stressful. Run by the nurse manager and liaison psychiatrist, it serves to identify special problems, difficult patients, and staff conflicts and facilitates their management.

Clearly, there is an interaction between the house officer, who uses a range of ways of adapting and coping, and the social environment. Actually, both personal resources (personality type and coping style) and interpersonal resources (social support and support of the work environment) counter the stresses. Kobasa (1979) described the "hardy" personality that copes well in stressful environments: one that uses commitment, control, and challenge in work.

Empirical research has found that business executives, lawyers, army officers, and others with a high number of stressors who had a strong sense of commitment to self and work, a more positive attitude toward change, and a greater belief in control over life reported fewer physical symptoms than those who did not have this personality style (Kobasa 1979; Kobasa 1982; Kobasa et al. 1982; Kobasa and Puccetti 1983). These aspects of personality and environmental factors led us to propose a study that assessed both contributions and the effect of an intervention upon them.

The MSKCC Intervention Study (1985–87)

GOALS OF STUDY

We proposed a study whose goals were to reduce stress in house officers by attempting to enhance information and communication, promote a sense of cohesiveness, and provide greater social support. We also proposed to encourage the house officers to behave in "hardy" ways that reinforced their sense of commitment and control at work and the challenge of their work. The goal to reduce staff stress was only a part of the outcome sought. The ultimate desired goal was to improve the human side of patient care by showing that a less stressed house staff would be perceived as more sensitive to patients' needs and would be better at communication. This model also recognized the need to keep the cost of any intervention as low as possible, use existing staff, and be easily implemented in other centers. We also recognized that to be acceptable, the intervention would have to be integrated into the existing unit structure and be directed toward the total social system of the unit. In order to assess whether house officers were more stressed while working on a cancer unit, we proposed to examine stress levels in their own hospital.

METHOD

This study was conducted by the Psychiatry Service in cooperation with the Departments of Medicine and Nursing over a two-year period. The first year was used to develop instruments to measure the particular stresses and to get baseline data. Kobasa led this effort, working with the chief resident and liaison psychiatrist. Two medical oncology units were

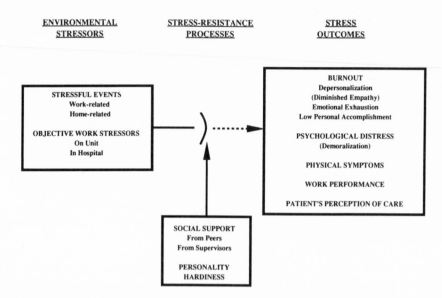

Figure 1. A model of stress and stress resistance in oncology staff.
(Adapted from Kobasa 1982.)

chosen because they were comparable in terms of types of patients, house staff, and nurses. They were randomized by a toss of a coin to experimental and control units in which the intervention was given over a twelve-month period.

Among the nurses and house staff, the baseline data included measurement of stress levels, burnout (Maslach 1982), psychological distress (demoralization), physical symptoms, and perceived stressors in their work. These data confirmed that house staff were high on two of the burnout measures, exhaustion and reduced empathy (depersonalization), as compared with other health care professionals and low (interns) to moderate (residents) on the sense of personal accomplishment burnout subscale. These data helped to identify components of the intervention.

The model of the study (figure 1) had three major components: (1) the environmental stressors related to work, objective work stressors, and personal stressors; (2) the outcome measures of impact on stress-related symptoms and patients' perception of care; and (3) the social system intervention. In terms of the work stresses, we asked about the workload, conflicts with attendings, cardiac arrests, resuscitations, the number of bone marrow transplants, the do not resuscitate orders, and the number of AIDS patients. On the personal side, we inquired about personal losses and illnesses.

We looked at physical and psychological symptoms as stress outcome variables, as well as the scales of the Maslach (1982) burnout inventory. Changes in work performance were explored by such questions as the number of needle sticks and the number of patient accidents and incidents. The unique aspect of this study, not usually investigated, was the effect on the patients' perception of care. Over an eighteen-month period (including three months before and after the intervention began and ended), 250 patients were interviewed about their perception of the house staff's behavior, their communication with the patients, and their sensitivity to the patients' needs.

In order to evaluate the effectiveness of the social system intervention, data were collected simultaneously on the experimental and control units from seventy house officers in a forty-five-minute questionnaire that tapped stress levels, hardiness, social support, physical and psychological symptoms, and burnout. These house officers were asked to fill out the questionnaire after they had worked on the medical oncology unit for four weeks and at two to four months after their oncology rotation when they were back on their own general medical units.

SOCIAL SYSTEMS INTERVENTION APPROACH

The intervention on the experimental floor focused on improving the level of information, communication, a sense of cohesiveness, and social support among staff working together by using a social systems approach (figure 2). The development of styles of coping to enhance "hardiness" was emphasized.

The specific components of the intervention were as follows:

1. New house staff were oriented to their new assignment prior to

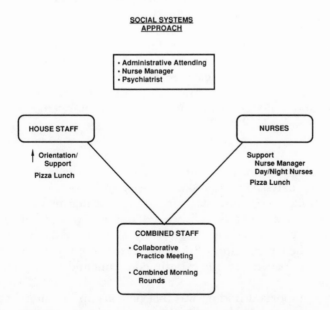

Figure 2. Social systems approach to stress intervention.

arrival for assignment. The physician coordinator and the project director met with each intern (and any resident who had not previously worked at MSKCC) at their parent hospital one to two weeks prior to beginning their assignment at MSKCC. Details about how to obtain a beeper, night call schedule, time and place to meet the chief resident, and types of patients they were going to be responsible for were discussed.

2. A weekly meeting was held by the physician coordinator with house officers to listen to their gripes and hassles at a pizza lunch. In addition, the physician coordinator was available to each house officer for at least ten minutes a week (and often more) to identify problems the house officers perceived in terms of patient or interstaff issues.

3. A weekly interdisciplinary unit meeting, the collaborative practice meeting, was attended by all disciplines on the unit: the administrative attending, the nurse manager, the liaison psychiatrist, nurses, house officers, social worker, and pharmacist. It provided a setting for interdisciplinary problems to be discussed and innovative administrative and educational procedures to be introduced. This meeting was chaired by the administrative attending and the nurse manager, both of whom were responsible for the administration of the unit as a whole. They were aware of morale, organizational, and administrative issues affecting the unit.

4. A weekly attending rounds for house officers was organized to review patient care issues which were particularly difficult to manage, such as do not resuscitate issues, legal problems, AIDS dementia and its management, demanding family members, management of an uncooperative patient, or management of interstaff problems. This permitted early identification by the physician coordinator of patients who may have later demonstrated psychological problems.

5. Morning rounds, previously separate, were combined for the house officers and the nurses so that treatment plans could be established for the day and all staff members were aware of the goals of other team members.

6. Assignment of an administrative attending to both the experimental and control floors allowed this attending to be incorporated in the intervention on the experimental floor.

RESULTS

Reported here are the preliminary findings from the house staff data. A more detailed analysis on house staff, nurses, and patients will be reported later. The number of house staff on both the experimental and control units who participated in this study was 70; of these, 40 were interns and 30 were residents. Of the participants, 23 were women and 47 were men. Two interns from the control unit refused to participate. Interviews were conducted with 137 patients on the experimental unit and 121 patients on the control unit.

The most important finding was that patients on the intervention unit expressed greater satisfaction with the "art" of the medical care given by house officers (interest, sensitivity, and compassion) than did patients on the control floor (p = .07), with a trend toward significance. Multiple regression analyses revealed that on the burnout subscale of emotional exhaustion, the more negative work stressors a house officer experienced, the greater the exhaustion reported. Interns reported more exhaustion than did residents and women more than men. The more support perceived as being given by the supervisor, the less reported exhaustion. Religion (none versus a little to a lot) was associated with less exhaustion among those who reported some religious beliefs.

On the personal accomplishment scale of the burnout inventory, a hardy personality style, increased supervisor support, and more peer cohesion correlated with a higher score. Examining the empathy scale of burnout, the house officer who reported some religious beliefs had higher scores on empathy. As negative work stressors increased, empathy decreased. As supervisor support increased, so did empathy. Men on the intervention unit had higher empathy scores than did men on the control unit.

On the demoralization scale, women scored higher than men. As negative work stress and social stress increased, so did demoralization scores. For those house officers with a hardy personality, there was less demoralization. As family stressors and social stressors increased, so did the number of physical symptoms. However, having a hardy personality style decreased the number of physical symptoms.

DISCUSSION OF FINDINGS

Among the findings, the trend toward a significantly more positive perception by patients of the human side of their care is important. Many uncontrolled factors, including a severe nursing shortage on the units in 1987, may have negatively affected our ability to show a more significant impact on patient care. Nevertheless, we feel that the data, even at this level, support our hypothesis that staff who are less hassled and who feel more supported are freer to give more sensitive care. A replication of the intervention study with more ideal overall staffing of both house staff and nurses might well show significant results. Such a study should be undertaken.

The other difference found between staff responses on the two units was that the male house officers on the intervention unit—but not the women—showed greater empathy. This supports our belief that a social systems approach that attempts to provide a generally more supportive environment has a salutary effect on staff. The absence of the effect in women may simply reflect small numbers; however, several prior studies have identified young women doctors as being more vulnerable to a sense of isolation and distress.

In terms of factors that impacted most significantly on burnout symptoms, greater negative work stressors (high number of patient deaths) correlated with greater exhaustion, demoralization, and diminished empathy. While the number of deaths cannot be reduced, the presence of a liaison psychiatrist and a supportive supervisor, along with sharing of the emotional burdens through such mechanisms as pizza lunches, clearly are important ways to mitigate the impact. In fact, good supervisor support, built into our intervention, was significantly associated with less burnout on all three subscales.

In keeping with findings in other stressful occupations, a hardy personality is a buffer that leads to enhanced personal accomplishment, fewer stress-related physical symptoms, and less demoralization,. Our intervention model sought to enhance hardiness by encouraging house staff to perceive new ways of controlling difficult situations, to plan ways to handle conflicting administrative procedures, and to feel a part of a group who could do their collective job well. The collaborative practice meeting also dealt constructively with enhancing supervisor support and a more informal camaraderie.

It comes as no surprise that personal stressors, such as an illness in someone close, were associated with more demoralization and more physical symptoms. This confirms our clinical impression that personal stressors make it more difficult to tolerate the stressors of the cancer work environment.

An unexpected finding based on the question "Do you consider yourself to be a religious person?" was the difference between those who responded with "not at all" versus "a little" to "extremely." Those who viewed themselves as at least somewhat religious reported lower levels of emotional exhaustion and higher levels of empathy for patients. The interpretation of this may be that they perceive dying and death in a more philosophical or religious vein. They may view the death of a patient and their own sense of personal loss in a different and more positive way. This would support findings that many patients tolerate advanced stages of cancer and death with equanimity. Similarly, parents who have lost a child with cancer have been found to adapt to their loss better when they have a philosophical or religious context in which to view the loss (Spinetta et al. 1981).

Finally, it is important to note that for all the stresses recounted and supports recommended, the rewards for most individuals in the health care professions outweigh the risks. It is, in the final analysis, a personal satisfaction in the work that keeps doctors working year after year. Peabody (1926) showed the quality required to survive, both personally and professionally, in a superb article written more than sixty years ago on patient care:

> What is spoken of as a "clinical picture" is not just a photograph of a man sick in bed; it is an impressionistic painting of the patient surrounded by his home, his work, his relations, his friends, his joys, sorrows, hopes and fears. . . . Thus the physician who attempts to take care of a patient while he neglects this [emotional] factor is as unscientific as the investigator who neglects to control all the conditions that may affect his experiment. . . . the treatment of disease imme-

diately takes its proper place in the larger problem of the care of the patient. . . . The treatment of a disease may be entirely impersonal; the care of a patient must be completely personal. . . . One of the essential qualities of the clinician is interest in humanity, for the secret of the care of the patient is in caring for the patient.

Summary

The oncology unit or cancer center carries with it basic stresses on the house officers who train there. Those who choose medicine are often individuals who are conscientious, feel responsibility heavily, and work long hours. Training reinforces these traits and, because it is physically and psychologically stressful, may result in symptoms of stress that, if unrecognized, can progress to a burnout syndrome and development of a psychiatric disorder in a vulnerable individual. Commonly seen is depression with dependence on alcohol or drugs; suicide is an outcome in some cases. Support for house officers is important, both as a group and as part of a meeting for all staff of a unit. Presented here is a model that not only reduces the negative impact of stress but also allows the patient to perceive the differences. Within cancer centers and, more broadly, medical centers there needs to be an increase in educational and supportive interventions that facilitate the house officer's ability to provide humane and compassionate patient care.

Dedication

It is a special privilege to contribute to this book in honor of Nancy Roeske. It is an honor not only because of the esteem in which we hold her and her memory, but because she became an "accidental" consultant on the work described in this chapter. Nancy sought out the psychiatric group on her admission to Memorial Sloan-Kettering Cancer Center in 1985. She rapidly became a participant observer in our study to improve the human side of care by reducing stresses on the staff. While in the hospital and on clinic visits, Nancy came to the meetings of the research team, offering suggestions and telling us of her own studies. Her enthusiasm, vitality, commitment, generosity, and sheer "goodness" encouraged our work. Her courage and remarkable equanimity in the face of illness were equally inspiring. This chapter is proudly dedicated to Nancy.

REFERENCES

Artiss, K. L., and Levine, A. S. (1973). Doctor-patient relation in severe illness: A seminar for oncology fellows. *New England Journal of Medicine*, 288, 1210–1214.
Bard, M. (1984). The cancer center as a social system. In *Current Concepts in Psycho-*

oncology: Syllabus for a Postgraduate Course (eds. M. J. Massie and L. M. Lesko). New York: Robert Gold Associates.

Borenstein, D. B., and Cook, K. (1982). Impairment prevention in the training years: A new mental health program at UCLA. *Journal of the American Medical Association*, 247, 2700–2703.

Cartwright, L. K. (1979). Sources and effects of stress in health careers. In *Health Psychology* (eds. G. C. Stone, F. Cohen, and N. E. Adler). San Francisco: Jossey Bass.

Fox, R. (1962). *Experiment Perilous*. Glencoe, Ill.: Free Press.

Friedman, R. C., Kornfeld, D. S., and Bigger, J. D. (1973). Psychological problems associated with sleep deprivation in interns. *Journal of Medical Education*, 48, 436–441.

Gaensbauer, T. J., and Mizner, G. L. (1980). Developmental stresses in medical education. *Psychiatry*, 43, 60–70.

Hall, R. C. W., Gardner, E. R., Perl, M., Stickney, S. K., and Pfefferbaum, B. (1979). The professional burnout syndrome. *Psychiatric Opinion*, 16, 12–17.

Holland, J. C. (1982). Psychological aspects of cancer. In *Cancer Medicine* (eds. J. F. Holland and E. Frei), 2d ed. Philadelphia: Lea and Febiger.

Holland, J. C., and Holland, J. F. (1985). A neglected problem: The stresses of cancer care on physicians. *Primary Care and Cancer (Oncology Rounds)*, 5, 16–22.

Hsu, K. and Marshall, V. (1987). Prevalence of depression and distress in a large sample of Canadian residents, interns and fellows. *American Journal of Psychiatry*, 144, 1561–1566.

Kobasa, S. C. (1979). Stressful life events, personality, and health: An inquiry into hardiness. *Journal of Personality and Social Psychology*, 37, 1–11.

Kobasa, S. C. (1982). Commitment and coping in stress resistance among lawyers. *Journal of Personality and Social Psychology*, 42, 707–717.

Kobasa, S. C., Maddi, S. R., and Kahn, S. (1982). Hardiness and health: A prospective study. *Journal of Personality and Social Psychology*, 42, 168–177.

Kobasa, S. C., and Puccetti, M. C. (1983). Personality and social resources in stress resistance. *Journal of Personality and Social Psychology*, 45, 839–850.

Maslach, C. (1979). The burnout syndrome and patient care. In *Stress and Survival: The Emotional Realities of Life-Threatening Illness* (ed. C. A. Garfield). St. Louis: C. V. Mosby.

Maslach, C. (1982). *Burnout: The Cost of Caring*. Englewood Cliffs, N.J.: Prentice-Hall.

McCue, J. D. (1982). The effects of stress on physicians and their medical practice. *New England Journal of Medicine*, 306, 458–463.

Millerd, E. J. (1977). Health professionals as survivors. *Journal of Psychiatric Nursing and Mental Health Services*, 15, 33–36.

Mount, B. M. (1986). Dealing with our losses. *Journal of Clinical Oncology*, 4, 1127–1134.

Peabody, F. W. (1926). The care of the patient. *Journal of the American Medical Association*, 88, 877–882.

Reuben, D. B. (1983). Psychologic aspects of residency. *Southern Medical Journal*, 76, 380–382.

Richards, A. I., and Schmale, A. H. (1974). Psychosocial conferences in medical oncology. *Annals of Internal Medicine*, 80, 541–545.

Ross, M. (1971). Suicide among physicians. *Psychiatry Medicine*, 2, 189–198.

Siegel, B., and Donnelly, J. C. (1978). Enriching personal and professional development: The experience of a support group for interns. *Journal of Medical Education*, 53, 908–914.

Small, G. (1981). House officer stress syndrome. *Psychosomatics*, 22, 860–869.

Smith, J. W., Denny, W. F., and Witzke, D. B. (1986). Emotional impairment in internal medicine house staff. *Journal of the American Medical Association, 255,* 1155–1158.

Spikes, J., and Holland, J. C. (1975). The physician's response to the dying patient. In *Psychological Care of the Medically Ill* (eds. J. J. Strain and S. Grossman). New York: Appelton-Century-Crofts.

Spinetta, J., Swarner, J., and Sheposh, J. (1981). Effective parental coping following death of a child from cancer. *Journal of Pediatric Psychology,* 6, 251–263.

Strain, J. J., and Hammerman, D. (1978). Ombudsmen (medical-psychiatric) rounds. *Annals of Internal Medicine,* 88, 550–555.

Vachon, M. L. S. (1987). *Occupational Stress in the Care of the Critically Ill, the Dying, and the Bereaved.* Washington, D.C.: Hemisphere.

Valko, R. J., and Clayton, P. J. (1975). Depression in the internship. *Diseases of the Nervous System,* 36, 26–29.

Weinstein, H. (1983). A committee on well-being of medical students and house staff. *Journal of Medical Education,* 58, 373–381.

Wise, T. N. (1977). Utilization of group process in training oncology fellows. *International Journal of Group Psychotherapy,* 27, 105–111.

Part Four

Physician Training

A SOCIOCULTURAL PERSPECTIVE

The final chapter in our volume, by Renée C. Fox, was originally delivered on March 31, 1989, at Princess Margaret Hospital in Toronto as the Philippa Harris Annual Psychosocial Lecture (established in memory of Ms. Harris, who died of cancer when she was twenty years old). In keeping with the conditions of this lecture series, an abridged version of Dr. Fox's contribution to this book appears in the Canadian journal *Humane Medicine*.

We have included her paper on "the perennial problem" of "training in caring competence" in this volume for several reasons. First, Dr. Fox generously acted as a reviewer for this book during the time that she was preparing her paper, and both the theme that she addresses and her reflections upon it were significantly influenced by the content of the contributions that she read. In addition, from the inception of her career as a sociologist of medicine, Dr. Fox has been continually involved as a "participant-observer" researcher and teacher in the process and problems of becoming a physician. In the opinion of the editors, the context and manner in which she considers the issues surrounding medical education make it a fitting conclusion to our volume.

There is also a more personal reason for incorporating a contribution from her in this book. Renée Fox and Nancy Roeske came to know each other when Nancy was a fourth-year medical student at Cornell University Medical College in New York City and Renée was a member of a team of social scientists affiliated with the Bureau of Applied Social Research of Columbia University who were conducting a series of studies in the sociology of medical education.* Renée's particular assignment involved four years of continuous, firsthand field research at Cornell Medical School. It was in this way that Nancy and she met, and very rapidly became colleagues and friends. Their relationship was both kindled and deepened by the fact that as a senior medical student, Nancy did an original study of the psychosocial experiences that polio patients and their families underwent. Renée,

*For a sociohistorical account of this research project, see Robert K. Merton, George Reader, and Patricia L. Kendall, eds., *The Student-Physician: Introductory Studies in the Sociology of Medical Education* (Cambridge, Mass.: Harvard University Press, 1957).

who had had polio at age 17, and her parents volunteered to be the initial "subjects" of the face-to-face interviews and life history–based inquiry that Nancy had designed. Nancy and Renée's medical school–born relationship not only lasted but was strengthened over the years by the mutual admiration that they had for each other's work and by the wellsprings of commitment out of which their work grew. We can certainly attest to the high esteem in which Nancy held Renée, whom she considered to be a major influence in her work. We have little doubt that had Nancy Roeske been able to choose a colleague to write the concluding chapter in a book honoring her career, that person would have been Renée Fox.

TWELVE

Training in Caring Competence

The Perennial Problem in North American Medical Education

RENÉE C. FOX

> . . . We must learn the science to practice
> the art. . . . Our competence makes room
> for the growth of our compassion, our hu-
> maneness.
>
> > —Samuel Shem, Introduction
> > to Dell's Tenth Anniversary
> > Edition of *The House of God*

> . . . [M]edical education has been changing
> constantly. Nevertheless the teaching/
> learning experience remains remarkably
> similar. . . . How can one explain this
> history of reform without change, of
> repeated modifications of the medical
> school curriculum that alter only very
> slightly or not at all the experiences of the
> critical participants, the students and the
> teachers?
>
> > —Samuel W. Bloom, "Structure
> > and Ideology in Medical Education:
> > An Analysis of Resistance to
> > Change," *Journal of Health and Social
> > Behavior* 29 (December 1988), p.
> > 295

In late December 1988, a number of American medical journals and
newspapers published feature articles summing up the findings of a
National Seminar on Medical Education that had been convened in No-

vember to consider how the clinical education of "the doctor of tomorrow" might be improved. The seminar's three-day meeting, which took place at the New York Academy of Medicine and was funded by the Josiah Macy Jr. Foundation, had been preceded by five months of interchange between its thirty-four participants, who included medical school deans and professors, hospital officials, and representatives of medical associations and relevant U.S. federal government agencies. In the materials that the working group issued to the press, their chairman, David E. Rogers, stated that "despite the diversity of the backgrounds and experiences of the participants, there was surprising unanimity of views about a number of important points," beginning with consensus about the "attributes" that "characterize our best physicians," and the importance of encouraging and strengthening these qualities in and through "the education of those becoming doctors." According to Rogers,[1] among the "points of general agreement" were the following:

> Our nation needs doctors with a broader and more sensitive view of the place and role of medicine in the larger society. . . .
>
> Our nation needs doctors who are more skillful in doctor-patient relationships. We should introduce a better blend of humanism and science into our health care institutions and the students they graduate.
>
> Modern physicians should pay more attention to health promotion, disease prevention, and the social, environmental, and emotional factors bearing on health.
>
> Both the physicians who graduate and the academic medical institutions that produce them should have a strong sense of social responsibility for the health and medical care rendered in their communities. It is of particular concern that inadequate funding of health care for the poor most severely affects those medical schools whose clinical and educational missions focus on service to indigent and minority groups. . . .

As I read these praiseworthy, collective affirmations, it was not Rogers's pleased surprise that I experienced as much as a rather dispirited sense of déjà vu. It occurred to me that this was essentially what the *Physicians for the Twenty-First Century* report published in 1984 by the Association of American Medical College's Project on the General Professional Education of the Physician and College Preparation for Medicine (GPEP) had also ringingly declared. I quote from the Introduction to that report:

> . . . The Panel's deliberations are rooted in the question of whether or not common attributes should characterize all physicians. Our answer is affirmative. We believe that every physician should be caring, compassionate, and dedicated to patients—to keeping them well and to helping them when they are ill. Each should be committed to work, to learning, to rationality, to science, and to serving the greater society. Ethical sensitivity and moral integrity, combined with equanimity, humility and self-knowledge, are quintessential qualities of all physicians. The ability to weigh possibilities and to devise a plan of action responsive to the personal needs of each patient is vital. Although every physician may not possess these ideal attributes in full measure, each physician is obligated to strive

to attain and maintain these attributes. Therefore, we affirm that the goal of the general professional education of physicians comprises both the acquisition of these attributes and the preparation for specialized education in medicine, and that these two purposes are not only compatible but also mutually support-ive. . . .[2]

But why should I be disheartened by the fact that two consecutive panels of distinguished medical spokespersons shared and articulated a holistic view of the good physician of today and tomorrow that placed as much emphasis on the emotional, interpersonal, environmental, social, and moral aspescts of what is involved in caring for illness, and promoting health, as on its more strictly biomedical components; that these experts insisted on the inherent compatibility of the multiple dimensions of doc-torhood, as well as on their essentialness; and that they used their authority to strongly urge that the process of medical education should enable physicians to "acquire values and attitudes that promote caring and concern for the individual and for society,"[3] along with the acquisition of scientific knowledge and technical skills? It is because throughout my entire career as a sociologist of medicine, from the early 1950s to the present, at periodic, closely spaced intervals, these kinds of formal, often quasi-official state-ments have been made by representatives of the medical profession, par-ticularly those involved in medical education. Each time they have contained virtually the same rediscovered principles and qualities of good physicianhood and medical care, the same concern over the degree to which these conceptions are being honored more in the breach than in practice, the same explanatory diagnoses of what accounts for these defi-ciencies, along with renewed dedication to remedying them through essen-tially the same exhortations and reforms. The perennial nature of this phenomenon is acknowledged in the Introduction and the Afterword of the 1984 AAMC/GPEP report, *Physicians for the Twenty-First Century:*

> . . . A review of past efforts to modify medical education reveals that most of the problems identified in the course of this project are not new. Institutions intermittently have changed their curricula, but unfortunately little progress has been made toward a fundamental reappraisal of how physicians are edu-cated. Thus, we do not claim novelty in the discovery of deficiencies. What we assert is the increasing urgency of finding appropriate remedies. . . .[4]

> . . . The Association of American Medical Colleges' Commission on Medical Education, appointed in 1925, identified problems in medical education not dissimilar to those that the Panel has pinpointed. . . . [This] underscores the need for dedicated leadership within our institutions if we are to accomplish in the last . . . years of this century what we so optimistically predicted 50 years ago.[5]

Although the language in which these concerns and affirmations have been expressed has varied somewhat from one decade to another, there is one preoccupation—one major theme—that is central to all of them: the importance of caring for and caring about patients with competence that is compassionate, and compassion that is competent. It is what Dr. Elizabeth Blackwell, a nineteenth-century leader in the movement to train women in medicine, eloquently termed "that intelligent sympathy with suffering which is a fundamental quality in the good physician."[6] The periodic invocation of the caring core of physicianhood has usually been accompanied by references to certain social and moral attitudes that physicians should ideally bring to their relationships with patients (sensitivity, empathy, responsiveness, equanimity, humility, integrity, and dedication foremost among them); by emphasis on the importance of preventive as well as therapeutic medicine; and by appeals to what has often been held up as the touchstone of physicians' commitment to the welfare of the larger society—their involvement in tending to the health and medical needs of those who are poor and disadvantaged.

I would like to devote the opportunity afforded me by the Philippa Harris Lecture to explore some of the factors associated with the persistent problem of fostering the development of caring competence in physicians and to consider the manner in which the medical profession has recurrently tried to deal with it, in and through the process of medical education. Although I do not claim to have the kinds of ideas that can definitively solve such a complex problem (or even spare us another ritualized cycle of discovering that it still exists), I hope that I can suggest a framework of reflection that is conducive to more insightful and effective ways of approaching it.

Dealing with Dichotomies

In our North American societies, the most fundamental challenges involved in training physicians to be caringly competent stem from nothing less than the imprint of Western thought upon our version of modern medicine. Out of this highly analytic, logico-rational way of thinking and viewing the world has come a chain of paired dichotomies, basic to our cultural tradition, that are also deeply institutionalized in both the cognitive and practicum structure of our medicine. These antithetically juxtaposed pairs include body vs. mind; thought vs. feeling; objective vs. subjective; explanation vs. understanding; material vs. spiritual; self vs. other; and individual vs. social, communal, and societal. In our medical educational curriculum, such polarities have found reified expression in the split conceptions of health and illness, their so-called biomedical as opposed to psychosocial components, and the sharp distinctions that are maintained between basic science and clinical aspects of medicine. They have even penetrated the subject matter and vocabulary of medical scientific fields such as immunology, with its "self" vs. "not-self" terms for identifying the body's ability to recognize "foreign" tissue.

So obdurate are these dichotomizing tendencies that they do not yield easily, if at all, to theoretical, empirical, or technological medical advances or to attempted reforms in medical education. This is illustrated in a rather ironic form by what psychiatrists have identified as one of the major challenges facing their discipline in the forthcoming century—namely, integrating the concepts of mind and brain. This was the recurrent theme at an October 1988 meeting on the "Next Steps That Will Revolutionize Psychiatry in the 21st Century."[7] According to the account of it written up in *Science:*

> . . . Participants agreed that psychiatrists need to combine the ever-increasing mass of information about the biological aspects of brain function and mental illness with the social, cultural, and psychological factors that also influence human behavior. . . . The obvious benefits of high technology for rapid diagnosis and drugs for specific illness notwithstanding, some foresee a struggle to keep the humanity in psychiatry. . . . [P]sychiatrists remind one another to maintain a broad, humanistic perspective and to integrate the basic, natural, and behavioral sciences in the clinical practice of medicine.[8]

As (Harvard Medical School) Professor of Psychiatry Leon Eisenberg astutely observed at this same meeting, although in the course of his own professional lifetime the conceptual framework of psychiatry has been turned upside down, its bedrock dichotomies have neither been altered nor bridged. In his words: "When I began as a medical student, psychiatry was brainless. The brain was not the object of study; it was seen as being in the head for ballast. That view has changed. But now psychiatry is getting mindless."[9]

Seen in cross-cultural perspective, the dualism of our medical thinking and our difficulties in breaking through it are distinctively and rather oddly Western. In non-Western societies and medical systems whose world views are more holistic than our own, there is no need for special fields, meetings, lectures, courses, and rhetoric to "remind" and teach medical students and practitioners that human beings have bodies and minds, and minds and brains that are dynamically interrelated; that ideally, the prevention, diagnosis, and treatment of illness should be approached in a "biopsychosocial" framework; that medicine is "both a science and an art"; that "the patient is a whole person"; or that "patients have families"—to use some of the clumsy, aphoristic phrases that we have coined in this connection.

What is as striking as the way that we have continued to be captives of our own dichotomies are the medical educational efforts that we have repeatedly made to surmount them. Each time, there have been curriculum reforms, triggered by still another *prise de conscience* about a too-great emphasis on the biological and technical aspects of medicine at the expense of what have variously and alternatively been called its psychological, social, cultural, interpersonal, behavioral, environmental, ethical, moral, and/or humanistic components. Sometimes these reforms have consisted of devising whole new programs, such as the wave of "Comprehensive Care" programs that were instituted in the 1950s or Harvard Medical School's so-called "New Pathways" program of the 1980s. Bringing student-physicians into earlier, more sustained relations with patients, locating more of their medical training in ambulatory care settings, increasing their opportunities to have collaborative contact with nurses and social workers, psychiatrists and social scientists, and requiring a period of community service as part of becoming a doctor have been key elements in a number of such reforms. The most recurrent pattern of all has been to inject designated new courses into the curriculum, as if they were intellectual magic bullets that could remedy the perceived dualism and imbalance in medical training. Over the course of the last three decades, from the 1950s through the 1980s, North American medical schools have moved *in seratim* from psychiatry, to psychosomatic medicine, to social and behavioral science, to community medicine, to bioethics, to the humanities in their search for such formulaic solutions.

Struggling with "Dehumanization" and "Brutalization"

There is a second major source of the difficulties involved in training physicians to develop and integrate competence that is at once scientific and technical, psychological and social, and moral, and to implement that multicompetence in an empathically caring way. This is what many commentators have described as the "dehumanizing," even "brutalizing" effects that our system of medical training can have on the men and women who undergo it.

In part, this phenomenon emanates from the encounters that medical students, interns, and residents have with the "human condition" and the "uncertainty" dimension of health, illness, and medicine.[10] Ruth Charon (a doctor and writer who is a faculty member at the College of Physicians and Surgeons of Columbia University), has movingly described some of the basic and transcendent aspects of the human condition, inherent in medical work, with which neophyte physicians must learn to deal:

> . . . Patients come to doctors for trivial or tragic problems. We occupy a peculiar place for them. We are the ones who diagnose and treat their physical problems, but we also stand for a level of the transcendent in their lives. We preside at scenes of human crisis—pain, loss, death, as well as joyous ones like birth and recovery. . . . [W]e are granted entrance into private, sometimes horrifying, often sad and always significant worlds. We are the interpreters for patients' dealings with dark and troubling events. We as physicians embody patients' hopes that they will live forever, and they expect that we can intercede with the gods or the fates when the time comes. We are the gatekeepers not only to services of subspecialists and fancy technology but also gatekeepers to the land of the living. . . . Because of the nature of the work we do with patients, we are in touch with deep levels of meaning in their lives. . . .[11]

Even before they start the clinical phases of their training, when they dissect a cadaver in the anatomy laboratory, for example, or participate in an autopsy, student-physicians "meet the mystery of life and the enigma of death in the form of a naked fellow human being who is laid out on a stainless steel table."[12] As soon as they begin their course work in physical diagnosis, they enter inner chambers of patients' bodies and of their "stories" and feelings. Through these experiences, charged with existential and metaphysical as well as biological and emotional significance, young doctors-in-becoming also undergo what I call "training for uncertainty." They learn in a variety of concrete, experienced ways that whatever they do as physicians will always be "accompanied by uncertainties that stem both from how much and how little they [personally] know, and how much is [and] is not known in the field of medicine."[13]

As they struggle, individually and collectively, to manage the primal feelings, the questions of meaning, and the emotional stress that the human condition and uncertainty aspects of their training evoke, medical students and house staff commonly develop certain ways of coping with them. Foremost among these socially patterned defense mechanisms are distancing themselves from their own feelings and from their patients through intellectual engrossment in the biomedical challenges of diagnosis and treatment, and participation in highly structured, in-group forms of medical humor. "Counterphobic and ironic, infused with bravado and self-mockery, often impious, defiant and macabre," this humor "characteristically centers on medical uncertainty, the limitations of medical knowledge, medical errors, and the side effects of medical and surgical interventions, the failure to cure, sex and sexuality, and, above all, death."[14] What young physicians are seeking is attainment of the measure of objectivity and equanimity that they need to navigate and do their work competently, without unduly undermining their capacity for empathy and compassion.[15] It is when they overshoot the mark and become hyper-detached, as many of them do, that the phenomenon called "dehumanization" occurs.

By and large, medical students and house staff are left to grapple with these experiences and emotions on their own. They are rarely accompanied, guided, or instructed in these intimate matters of doctorhood by mature teachers and role models. The relations of clinical faculty and attending physicians with students and house staff are generally too sporadic and remote for that.

What has been termed the "brutal and brutalizing" process to which physicians-in-training are subject has usually been associated with the years of internship and residency. It has been critically described in the plethora of medical journal articles about the "hardships" of internship and residency, and in the corpus of memoirs written by young physicians, portraying what they underwent during their house staff years—particularly how, as one of them expressed it, they battled for "survival as a human being."[16] These accounts identify several interconnected sources of what Samuel Shem (author of *The House of God,* the most renowned of the book-length narratives about the house staff phase of training) calls this "cycle of brutality."[17]

Foremost among the conditions that these writings identify as threats to the humanity and humaneness of interns and residents is what is described as the "ordeal" of their "on-call" schedule. At its 1987 annual meeting, the American Medical Association (AMA) officially acknowledged that this "exhausting and often onerous schedule" of "long hours and no sleep" can have serious negative consequences both for the technical competence and the human quality of the care that such physically and emotionally fatigued young physicians deliver to their hospitalized patients.[18] The time had come to address this problem, announced the AMA delegates, thereby joining their voices with all the medical professional spokespersons over the years who have insisted that the "brutal on-call schedule" must be mitigated, if not completely abolished. But, as the AMA delegates recognized, these ardors of house officer training constitute an "historical pattern endured by generations of physicians"[19] that is highly resistant to change. It continues to be powerfully supported by the conviction of many physicians that such rites-of-passage challenges have indispensable value in preparing young initiates into the medical profession for the highest, most exigent responsibilities of their vocation. These sentiments were vociferously expressed, for example, in what the editors of the *Journal of the American Medical Association (JAMA)* referred to as the "avalanche . . . of commentary" they received from physician-readers responding to an article by Norman Cousins, which the *JAMA* had published, entitled "Internship: Preparation or Hazing?" In this article, Cousins asserted that: "The custom of overworking interns has long since outlived its usefulness. It doesn't lead to the making of better physicians. It is inconsistent with the public interest. It is not worthy of the medical profession."[20] A sizable number of letters to the editor written to *JAMA* about this article came from physicians who strongly disagreed with what Cousins said, on the moral grounds that "aspiring physicians should be prepared to undergo a reasonable degree of hardship in their ascent to a profession built upon a tradition of personal sacrifice. Since medicine is dedicated to healing and the alleviation of human suffering, the training of physicians should emphasize the subordination of their personal comforts and perquisites."[21]

There is another, serious kind of stress from which interns and residents suffer, which they believe corrodes their ability to be caring and compassionate. It issues from house staff's intensive, minute-to-minute contact with what often seems to them to be the unending procession of hospitalized patients for whose physical, psychological, and social problems they can offer no satisfactory solution and little relief. The "front-line" nature of interns' and residents' exposure to and responsibility for taking care of so many patients who personify both the limits of our medicine and the ills of our society takes an emotional toll on them. Among the experiences that are hardest on them—that make them feel especially inadequate, perplexed, frustrated, angry, and fearful—are encounters with patients who are very poor and battered by their deprived and degrading environment; who are homeless and gravely ill, physically and/or mentally; who are alcoholics or drug addicts; who are elderly and isolated from the human community because they are mentally impaired by Alzheimer's disease or are alone in the world; who have contracted AIDS; or whose illnesses and suffering are being prolonged or made worse, rather than improved, by the advanced medical treatment they are receiving.

In this connection, it is edifying to take note of one of the classic defense mechanisms that house staff physicians collectively develop: the bitterly humorous, often scathing in-group vocabulary that they invent and use as "backstage" labels for patients. In analyzing the results of the study that they conducted of when and why the internal medicine residents in one university hospital applied the perjorative label *gomer* to patients, Deborah B. Leiderman and Jean-Anne Grisso (young physicians with social science training) pointed out that

> gomers were patients whose illnesses and management posed special frustra-tions for resident physicians. Gomers suffered irreversible mental deteriora-tion; their illnesses were complex and intractable; they were unable to resume normal adult social roles; and they had no place to go after discharge. . . .
>
> The gomer patient who deteriorates in the hospital, whose illness is unlikely to be significantly improved by medical treatment, who has no concerned family to place him in a meaningful social network and confer personhood as opposed to mere patienthood upon him, confronts resident physicians with . . . pro-found threats to their ideals of themselves as physicians. . . .[22]

Interns and residents attest that the great physical and emotional de-mands placed upon them and the resulting state of chronic sleep depriva-tion, distress, and desensitization to others in which they find themselves are made all the worse by their sense of aloneness and of virtual abandon-ment by senior-physician teachers and models. "The important thing about brutalization is that we were alone," Samuel Shem declared (at a workshop/ symposium on "The Physician as Writer"): "There was nobody there. The phrase that comes to mind is: 'Be with the patient.' The value of medicine is being with the patient. [But] if no one is with you, then you can't be with anybody."[23]

Where Are the Teachers? And How Are They Teaching?

The physical, intellectual, and interpersonal absence of dedicated teachers and clinical supervisors is keenly felt by interns, residents, and medical students alike. The phenomenon to which they allude is more than a state of mind or a set of attitudes on their part. It is an objective fact that in current American medical education, in many—probably most—medical school and house staff settings, such teachers and teaching are minimally present.

This is a long-standing problem in medical education. Particularly since World War II, medical schools and academic health centers have increasingly emphasized the importance of faculty involvement in biomedical research and specialty practice at the expense of teaching. In the 1980s, this situation has worsened, so that despite the enormous size of medical school faculties and clinical departments, fewer and fewer senior physicians are now involved in serious teaching. As I have stated elsewhere:

> Senior faculty have been taken away from the teaching act because they are heads of departments and groups that have become as large as whole medical schools used to be. They are consumed by managerial and budgetary functions [including the obligation to generate their own salaries through clinical practice], and [they] do not walk the corridors of learning with their students. Medical students are being taught by house staff, and house staff are being taught by house staff.[24]

Returning to the teaching of medicine "after a 15-year hiatus" (during which time he served as president of the Robert Wood Johnson Foundation), David E. Rogers[25] expressed "dismay" over the degree to which medical education has "drifted off track" in this regard. "The dimensions of the problem," he writes, "are apparent in Hiliard Jason and Jane Westberg's disquieting 1982 study, *Teachers and Teaching in Medical Schools* . . . based on a survey of several thousand full-time faculty. . . . A few findings from this study tell the tale":

> 60 percent of full-time faculty spent less than 5 hours per week teaching. . . . the majority felt that the kinds of attitudes developed by students about what it means to be a physician, and their skills in dealing with ambiguity were not very important. . . . a scant 3 percent of the medical-school faculty polled felt that community service was of any importance whatsoever, and most of them actually felt that such service detracted from medical school activities.[26]

Even when faculty and attending physicians are present, the chief pedagogical methods that they use often have the effect of distancing students, interns, and residents from both the science and the clinical skills of medicine, from their teachers, and ultimately from patients. In David Rogers's words:

> . . . [T]oo many faculty members are simply stuffing students with the details of their own basic science or specialty. . . . We've tended to forget that the sum of the parts does not necessarily make a whole—at least not a whole doctor. We are force feeding students with up to 8 hours of lectures a day, denying them the time to explore learning on their own. . . . Gone are the go-at-your-own-pace problem-solving sessions, the informal after-hours get-togethers with faculty, and the leisurely laboratory work where students got to know faculty and learn more about the personal qualities of those who taught them.[27]

Sherman M. Mellinkoff, a professor on the faculty of the University of California in Los Angeles School of Medicine, says:

In most places, the student and the teacher spend less time with patients and more time with blackboards and lantern slides. Patients have almost vanished from "grand rounds," which are now lectures—often very good ones. "Teaching rounds" for medical students may be combined with the "business rounds" of residents, moving swiftly from bed to bed, sometimes over several floors, with brief discussions in the corridors. Other teaching rounds may be like small grand rounds, conducted mainly in a conference room, not at the bedside, in which the patient's illness, more than the patient is discussed in detail. . . . Ambulatory patients, with whom students in many medical schools used to spend almost a year, are usually seen very little or not at all in the study of internal medicine. . . . The patients that are available for teaching, inside or outside the hospital, more often present problems of management than of diagnosis. Less often, the student sees problems requiring front-line analysis, before biopsy and before CT scanning. . . . From many of their teachers and from the hospital records, students receive the answers to a large number of questions they did not generate. Facts surround the students without vivid connections to their patients' stories.[28]

Mellinkoff recognizes that "many [of these] complaints about current medical education are not new" and that some of them were identified more than fifty years ago by medical teachers of the stature of William Osler. He contends nonetheless that although they have "by no means become irretrievably separated," the goal of medical education—which is "to produce the physicians we would like to see if we were sick," and the "direction the educational process is [now] taking—[moving] increasingly toward the creation of an efficient, specialized staff member of a procedure-oriented care facility . . . are drifting apart."[29] He also implies that conveying the kind of "respect for the art of medicine" that does not entail "undervaluing science in medicine or failing to support and teach it enthusiastically," along with "respect for science," that does not "mean pretending a faint hauteur toward the craft of medicine confers upon anyone . . . intellectual grandeur," has become more problematic in medical teaching in recent years.[30]

And so we return full-circle to the dichotomies inherent in our medical culture and the larger world view of which it is a part—dichotomies that, in disjoining the art and science of medicine, also pull asunder its technical competence and empathic caring.

Reasoning toward Remedies

It is clear that the problems of training in caring competence that I have identified are associated with ways of thought, shared values, beliefs and sentiments, modes of organization, and patterns of behavior, rooted in our society, which have been institutionalized in distinctive, tenacious forms in our medicine and our process of medical education. This has contributed not only to the perennialness of these problems but also to the fact that the same relatively ineffective solutions to them have been proposed and enacted again and again.

During the interval of time that elapses between each new wave of medical educational attempts to improve these dimensions of training and socializing physicians, a certain amount of collective backsliding and forgetting seems to take place. This has led, in many instances, to the reinstitutionalization of what has been tried before. A recent example of this medical-educational equivalent of reinventing the wheel can be found in the following "suggestions for overcoming shortcomings" that were made by the Josiah Macy Jr. Foundation National Seminar in Medical Education:

> The education of future doctors should be an *institutional*, not a *departmental* function. [Italics are those of the seminar report.] Any significant changes in clinical education at a medical school will require the creation of a specific centralized education unit with recognized responsibility and authority to develop the basic curriculum. Medical student teaching must be recognized and honored by faculty in its own right—with stature, and with legitimacy for appointment and promotion, equal to that given research productivity and clinical excellence. . . . Substantial amounts of clinical teaching . . . should be moved to ambulatory settings. . . . If the social sensitivity of physicians is to be improved, the nation and its medical schools should consider requiring a period of community service for students as part of becoming a doctor. . . .[31]

It is noteworthy that neither the great scientific and technological advances in medical knowledge, clinical methods, and therapy that have occurred since World War II nor the major social and economic changes that have taken place in our system of health care delivery have significantly altered the manifestations and the underpinnings of the training in caring competence problem. Indeed, there are certain ways in which these advances and changes have reinforced the problem. For instance, the advent of the "biological revolution" and the preeminence of molecular biology in medicine that it has brought in its wake have deepened the split between basic scientific and clinical medicine, between micro- and macro-levels of medically relevant observation and analysis, and, above all, between the biological and nonbiological aspects of medicine. The kind of scientific determinism and reductionism that characterize molecular biology and the moral, social, and metaphysical assumptions that are coded into them have played a powerful latent role in this regard. Within this at-once scientific and philosophical framework, as sociologist Howard L. Kaye points out:

> . . . [C]ulture is reduced to biology; biology, to the laws of physics and chemistry at the molecular level; mind, to matter; behavior, to genes; organism, to program; the origin of species, to macromolecules; life, to reproduction. . . . The reductionism . . . represents both a research strategy (one that has been spectacularly successful), and something more: a world view. . . .[32]

In this perspective, much that was previously considered to be other or more than biological—including psychological, social, and cultural aspects of health, illness, and medicine—are biologized, and nonbiological factors are relegated to a residual category of lesser importance. Along with the penetrating properties of new forms of medical technology, the power of the microview of molecular biology has carried medicine further away from a holistic outlook. In the words of nurse Sallie Tisdale: "Our eye gets finer and finer every day, drawing us down until we are looking at smaller and smaller pieces of the whole. We ride it down the laser and scope and scanner, until we sit at the side of the cell and try to extrapolate from it the rest of the person."[33] In Tisdale's opinion, this is "a great relinquishment."[34]

As for the goal of teaching clinical medicine with equally balanced, reciprocal respect for its science and its art, educators such as Sherman Mellinkoff contend that this, too, has been made more difficult by the interplay of certain scientific, technological, social, and economic developments in the United States:

> Teaching hospitals and allied institutions have been made vastly more expensive to build and operate by a variety of factors, including scientific and technologic advances, measures designed to rectify historical inequities such as the low salaries of nurses, the failure to work out adequately rational and moral mechanisms for ensuring medical care for all who need it while not squandering resources on the prolongation of death, the population surge among the aged, and competition for money and talent by profit-driven corporations. Escalations in the fractions of the gross national product spent on medical care under these circumstances have given rise to blunt cost-containment efforts. These sometimes manage simultaneously to be unsuccessful, harmful to the spirit and quality of medical care, and damaging to medical education, especially at hospitals caring for the poor.[35]

In light of the interconnections that exist between important social and cultural patterns in our society and its institutions (including our science) and the problem of effectively training physicians to integrate competence and caring in their treatment of patients, it is hardly surprising that this has proven to be such a difficult and complex task. Nevertheless, we have continually failed to take the nonmedical factors that are inside as well as outside our medicine sufficiently into account, and we have consistently expected panacea-like results from rather simple and mechanistically implemented educational reforms. The epitome of such reforms has been the parachuting of courses in behavioral science, bioethics, human values, and the like into the medical curriculum, as if they were automatic and interchangeable promoters of humane and compassionate medical care.[36]

When I say that there are no facile solutions and that we should not suppose that there are, I do not mean this to be a counsel of resignation. I am not arguing for withdrawal from the task of trying to find better ways of interconnecting the scientific, technical, and attitudinal aspects of physicianhood in the medical educational process and of conveying them in their wholeness to the women and men becoming doctors. Nor am I suggesting that nothing of consequence can be done to improve training in caring competence without deep-structure changes in all of our medicine and science, in the macro-organization of our society, and in the quintessences of our culture and world view.

However, I do think that it makes a difference that is practical as well as theoretical to consider what I have called the "perennial problem" in American medical education within a larger sociocultural framework. For example, more detailed awareness by medical faculty of how the concepts, terminology, and methods of biomedicine are imprinted with dichotomies inherent in our cultural way of thought could provide them with new recognition of some of the bioscientific contexts in the curriculum where they are inadvertently teaching medical students and house staff to split competence from caring.

The kind of epistemological analysis that Yale Professor of Medicine and Epidemiology Alvan R. Feinstein has made of how "the devout reverence for hard data" that prevails in biomedicine produces "dehumanized science in patient care,"[37] has great value of this sort, too. The "'hard data' creed," Feinstein explains, often leads to the omission of so-called "soft" variables from the conduct of clinical research, and the way its findings are reported and taught:

> Since all of the uniquely human phenomena of patients are expressed in soft clinical data, the exclusion of such data creates a biostatistical clinical science that is deliberately dehumanized. The results that emerge from the trials do not contain information about the things that a practicing doctor and a patient might want to know in choosing a treatment. . . . The clinical science that emerges is hard and reliable, but is unsatisfactory as a guide to clinical practice because of its dehumanization. The investigators have systematically excluded the distinctly human clinical features that distinguish the practice of medicine from an abstract exercise in statistics.[38]

Sociologist Renée R. Anspach has made a comparable analysis of the language that interns and residents use in their formal presentations of case histories and of the implicit, unintentional consequences this medical discourse may have for the way of thought and the values they learn.[39] Anspach points out that case presentations are not only an important part of the work routine of house staff; in addition, because they are "self-presentations . . . delivered before superordinates," they are "instrument(s) for professional socialization."[40] Basing her analysis on the language of case presentations made by house staff in two intensive care nurseries and an obstetrics and gynecology service, Anspach found that "many of the values and assumptions" in the language they employed "contradict[ed] the explicit tenets of medical education." Most particularly, the medical discourse both reflected and created a "world view" that "emphasize[d] science, technology, teaching and learning at the expense of interactions with patients." In this view,

> biological processes exist apart from persons, observations can be separated from those who make them, and the knowledge obtained from measurement instruments has a validity independent of the persons who use and interpret this diagnostic technology. Inasmuch as presenting a case history is an important part of medical training, those who use the language of case presentation may be impelled to adopt an unquestioning faith in the superior scientific status of measurable information and to minimize the import of the patient's history and subjective experience.[41]

Anspach's and Feinstein's interpretive analyses invite us to consider the possibility that medical educators have paid too little attention to the effects that the cognitive content of medicine, the conceptions of science on which it is based, and the forms in which its knowledge is presented have on the attitudes, values, and beliefs that medical students, interns, and residents develop—especially those that are relevant to their physicianly competence to care. If this is true, then it seems to me that it might be worthwhile for physicians-in-training to have a systematic opportunity to explore the social and cultural matter embedded in the sciences they are studying, through courses in the philosophy, sociology, or intellectual history of medical science. It is an option that might be particularly appropriate during the first two years of medical school, while students are more immersed in the basic sciences than in the clinical practice of medicine. It might even be more appropriate than the courses in behavioral science and bioethics that are usually scheduled at this point in the curriculum and are generally focused on what are referred to as the "psychosocial" or "humanistic" aspects of medicine, in sharp contradistinction to its science.

It also seems to me that it would be both instructive and useful for medical educators to be more cognizant of the social and cultural as well as the psychological origins of the collective defense mechanisms that medical students and house staff physicians characteristically develop in the course of their training, more perceptive about the sociomedical situations out of which these group-patterned devices grow, and more thoughtful about their implications for the humane competence of the young women and men learning to be doctors under their tutelage. In discussing these shared ways of coping, I have implied here, as I have elsewhere, that because the work that physicians do confronts them with "basic human condition-associated stresses and dilemmas" inherent in medicine, they cannot "go naked" into it. "In order to do this sort of work, and do it well, they must develop intellectual and emotional 'clothing' that provides them with some degree of detachment and protection."[42] But does this necessarily mean that the mutual ways of coming to terms with these aspects of caring for patients that neophyte physicians adopt are inevitable—the only viable coping mechanisms that are available to them? For example, are the self-protective medical humor and the "gomer phenomenon," which I have described and located in the training sequence, unavoidable? Are there no other psychosocial means that developing young physicians can employ to deal with the disease and death, pain and suffering, injustice and tragedy that they encounter in their work, and with its medical uncertainties and limitations? And is there nothing that medical faculty and attending physicians can do to help the women and men they are teaching to find ways of coping that would enable them to stay in more open, feeling contact with their own humanity and that of their patients?

Virtually all the studies of medical education published by sociologists over the past three decades and the personal accounts of the process written by young physicians who have passed through it highlight the interrelationships that exist between the stresses of learning to be a doctor, the ways of coming to terms that medical students and house staff not only adopt but also institutionalize in their collective culture, and the problems of emerging from medical training with humane values, caring skills, and the capacity to put them into practice in the treatment of patients. And yet, when medical educators come together to plan or reform curriculum and training programs, they rarely speak of such matters or take them into account. I believe that it could have both general and specific educational value if they did. For example, a more felicitous ordering and timing of the experiences to which medical students and house staff are exposed in the training process might be arranged. In addition, new, organized opportunities might be designed for neophyte physicians to identify and analyze their shared stresses and modes of coping with them, in ways that could have both didactic and therapeutic value for them personally and in their relations with patients.

This brings us back once more to the questions "Where are the teachers? And how are they teaching?" that I posed earlier; to the complex attitudinal and organizational conditions that have, in effect, subtracted so many of them from in situ involvement with student-physicians, interns, and residents; and to the baseline fact that unless the teachers return to first-hand teaching, even the most cleverly insightful schemes for improving training in caring competence will surely fail.

I have not proposed any sweeping solutions to this very basic and persistent problem of medical education. However, I hope that by casting it in a somewhat different sociocultural framework than has ordinarily been brought to bear upon it, I have at last suggested some approaches to "reforming the reforms"[43] that have repeatedly been applied to the goal of fostering caring competence in future physicians.

NOTES

I am grateful to Judith P. Swazey for her helpfully critical reading of this paper.

1. David E. Rogers, "Clinical Education and the Doctor of Tomorrow: An Agenda for Action." Final chapter from Proceedings of the Josiah Macy Jr. Foundation National Seminar of Medical Education, "Adapting Clinical Medical Education to the Needs of Today and Tomorrow," eds. Barbara Gastel and David E. Rogers (New York Academy of Medicine, November 1988), in press.

2. Steven Muller, Introduction, *Physicians for the Twenty-First Century.* Report of the Panel on the General Professional Education of the Physician and College Preparation for Medicine (Washington, D.C.: Association of American Medical Colleges, 1984), pp. xi–xii.

3. Conclusion, *Physicians for the Twenty-First Century,* p. 1.

4. Muller, Introduction, *Physicians for the Twenty-First Century,* p. xiv.

5. John A. D. Cooper, Afterword, *Physicians for the Twenty-First Century,* pp. 35–36.

6. Elizabeth Blackwell, "Erroneous Method of Medical Education," in *Essays in Medical Sociology,* 2, ed. Elizabeth Blackwell (New York: Arno Press, 1891/1972), p. 43.

7. This meeting, held October 7 to 10, 1988, in New York City, was sponsored by the Department of Psychiatry and Behavioral Sciences of the New York Medical College.

8. Deborah M. Barnes, "Psychiatrists Psych Out the Future," *Science,* 242 (November 18, 1988), pp. 1013–1014.

9. Quoted in ibid.

10. See, Renée C. Fox, "Training for Uncertainty," in *The Student-Physician: Introductory Studies in the Sociology of Medical Education,* eds. Robert K. Merton, George Reader, and Patricia L. Kendall (Cambridge, Mass.: Harvard University Press, 1957), 207–241; and Renée C. Fox, "The Human Condition of Health Professionals," Distinguished Lecturer Series (Durham: University of New Hampshire, 1980). The University of New Hampshire Lecture has been reprinted in the second, enlarged edition of Renée C. Fox, *Essays in Medical Sociology: Journeys into the Field* (New Brunswick, N.J.: Transaction Books, 1988), 572–587.

11. Rita Charon, "To Listen, to Recognize," *Pharos* (Fall 1986), p. 12.

12. Fox, "The Human Condition of Health Professionals," p. 13.

13. Ibid., p. 16.

14. Ibid., pp. 23–24.

15. Harold I. Lief and Renée C. Fox, "Training for 'Detached Concern' in Medical Students," in *The Psychological Basis of Medical Practice,* eds. Harold I. Lief, Victor F. Lief, and Nina R. Lief (New York: Harper and Row, 1963), 12–35.

16. Samuel Shem, Introduction, *The House of God,* Tenth Anniversary Edition (New York: Dell, 1988), no pagination.

17. Ibid.

18. Christine Hinz, "Scheduling, Supervision of Residents To Be Examined," *American Medical News,* July 3–10, 1987, p. 9.

19. Ibid.

20. Norman Cousins, "Internship: Preparation or Hazing?" *Journal of the American Medical Association,* 245, no. 4 (January 23/30, 1981), 377.

21. "Internship: Physicians Respond to Norman Cousins," *Journal of the American Medical Association,* 246, no. 19 (November 13, 1981), 2141–2144. The quotation is taken from Norman Cousins's summary of and response to these recurrent themes ("Norman Cousins Responds," p. 2144).

22. Deborah B. Liederman and Jean-Anne Grosso, "The Gomer Phenomenon," *Journal of Health and Social Behavior,* 26 (September 1985), 222–232.

23. Judith C. Watkins, edited transcript of a symposium on "The Physician as Writer," held under the auspices of the Cooper Institute for Advanced Studies in Medicine and the Humanities and organized and chaired by Renée C. Fox, Naples, Florida, November 10–12, 1988, p. 157.

24. "Medical Uncertainty: An Interview with Renée C. Fox," *Second Opinion*, 6 (November 1987), p. 104.

25. David Rogers is now Walsh McDermott University Professor of Medicine at the New York Hospital–Cornell Medical Center. Before becoming President of the Robert Wood Johnson Foundation, he was Chairman of Medicine at Vanderbilt University and Dean of the Faculty of Medicine at Johns Hopkins University.

26. David E. Rogers, "Prescription for Medical Education," *Issues in Science and Technology* (Winter 1988–1989), pp. 31–32.

27. Ibid., p. 31.

28, Sherman M. Mellinkoff, "The Medical Clerkship," *New England Journal of Medicine*, 317, No. 17 (October 22, 1987), p. 1089.

29. Ibid.

30. Ibid., p. 1090.

31. Rogers, "Clinical Education and the Doctor of Tomorrow."

32. Howard L. Kaye, *The Social Meaning of Modern Biology: From Social Darwinism to Sociobiology* (New Haven, Conn.: Yale University Press, 1986), pp. 55–56.

33. Sallie Tisdale, *The Sorcerer's Apprentice: Inside the Modern Hospital* (New York: McGraw Hill, 1986), p. 245.

34. Ibid.

35. Mellinkoff, "The Medical Clerkship," p. 1091.

36. At the time I was writing this part of the Philippa Harris Lecture, I received an announcement in the mail about a forthcoming American Board of Medical Specialties conference on the "Teaching and Evaluation of Humanism" that typified this approach. According to the notice, the morning session of the conference would highlight "The Importance of Humanism in the Physician," "How to Teach Humanism in Residents," and "How to Evaluate Humanism in Residents."

37. Alvan R. Feinstein, "Hard Science, Soft Data, and the Challenges of Choosing Clinical Variables in Research," *Clinical Pharmacology and Therapeutics*, 22, no. 4 (October 1977), p. 4901.

38. Ibid., p. 4903.

39. Renée R. Anspach, "Notes on the Sociology of Medical Discourse: The Language of Case Presentation," *Journal of Health and Social Behavior*, 29, no. 4 (December 1988), 357–375.

40. Ibid., p. 372.

41. Ibid.

42. Fox, "The Human Condition of Health Professionals," p. 35.

43. For articulating the need to reform the reforms that have been attempted in medical education, I am indebted to Robert H. Ebert and Eli Ginzberg's article "The Reform of Medical Education," published in a special supplementary issue of *Health Affairs*, 7 (1988), pp. 5–38.

Index

Acquired immune deficiency syndrome (AIDS): physicians and loss, 6; psychiatric illness, 28; students and communication, 66; students and prejudice, 95

Admissions, university: communication skills, 55; student population, 96

Adults: psychobiology of loss and separation, 9–10

Age: disease onset, 14–16; students and communication, 60–61; student population, 96

Albany Medical College: faculty development, 161

Alcohol and alcoholism: bereavement, 11; recognition and diagnosis, 37–38; Dartmouth Medical School, 152, 168–69

Alexithymia: psychology of somatizing patients, 31

Allergies: food and psychiatric illness, 28

Allopathic medicine: history of medical education, 131

American Association of Medical Colleges: problem-based learning, 147; faculty development, 157, 160–61

American Board of Internal Medicine: physicians and humanism, 107

American Board of Orthopaedic Surgeons: medical education research, 162

American Heart Association: faculty research, 160

American Medical Association (AMA): house staff and working hours, 206

American Psychiatric Association: mental health services and cost of general medical care, 36

Animals: mother-infant bond and health, 5; experimental studies of separation, 7–8; premature separation and disease, 13; separation and disease onset, 16–19

Anorexia nervosa: psychobiological makeup of patient, 14; endocrine system and age-related change, 15

Anxiety: chest pain and psychiatric illness, 27

Arthritis, rheumatoid: autoimmune factors and bereavement, 14

Art: bacteriological revolution and medicine, 120–21

Artists: teaching of physicians, 92

Association of American Medical Colleges. *See* GPEP Report

Asthma: predisposition and bereavement, 14

Attitudes: physicians, 72–75; students and educational environment, 129; faculty development, 157

Atypical somatoform disorder: psychiatric syndrome, 30

Authority: physician and patient, 55, 57; changing role of physician, 73–74

Bacteriology: science and medicine, 120–21; Blackwell on vivisection, 122

Balint group: Dartmouth Medical School, 152

Barrows, Howard: problem-based learning, 142

Behavioral sciences: curriculum, 75–77; influence and medical schools, 83

Bereavement: health effects, 5; choice of disease following, 13–14. *See also* Loss

Biochemistry: impact of neurochemical revolution, 91

Biology: molecular and medicine, 210–11

Blackwell, Elizabeth: women in medicine, 120; views on medical education and practice, 121; image of medical scientist, 121–22; research and education, 122; gender dichotomy, 126; caring and physicians, 202

Blood pressure: separation and development of high, 16–17

Body: as machine, 4; disturbance of image and psychiatric illness, 29

Bowman Gray Medical School: problem-based learning, 147

Brain: age and disease onset, 15–16; catecholamine and nucleoprotein and separation, 19; neurochemical revolution, 91

Briquet's syndrome: somatization disorder, 30

Broomall, Anna: obstetrics education, 123–24; as teacher, 126

Bureaucracy: doctor/patient relationship, 106

Burn-out: empathy and communication, 63; oncology house staff, 185–86, 191

Cancer: technology and treatment of patients, 164. *See also* Oncology

Cardiac surgery: students and communication, 67. *See also* Heart disease

Caring: physician and competence, 202

Case Western Reserve University: innovation and educational environment, 132; integration of basic sciences and clinical medicine, 141; organ system based curriculum, 141, 170; family clinic program, 150; faculty development, 154; curriculum innovation, 157–58; success of innovation, 166–67

Catecholamine: disturbances and separation, 19

Chest: pain and psychiatric illness, 26–27

Children: role of pediatrician, 175–76

Circadian rhythms: age and disease onset, 16
Civil War: chest pain and psychiatric illness, 26–27
Class: somatization, 32
Cleveland, Emmeline: as teacher, 126
Coma: communication, 64
Communication: research on problems in education, 55–59; students and sociocultural factors, 59–62; students and need for good, 62–63, 78; students and suggested solutions, 63–68; skills and medical education, 68–70; importance and approach, 92–93; innovations in course offerings, 137–38
Community: educational innovation and learning experiences, 148–54
Compassion: physicians and body as machine, 4; premedical school experience, 96; commitment of medical profession, 107–108
Competency: faculty development, 162–65
Computer: physicians and learning skills, 78–79
Computer-aided instruction (CAI): medical education, 136
Conversion disorder: psychiatric syndrome, 30
Coping: programs and medical students, 138–40; training of caringly competent physicians, 213–14
Cornell University Medical College: communication skills program, 64; student attitudes and educational environment, 129
Cosmetic surgery: body image and psychiatric illness, 29
Cost: general medical care and mental health services, 35–36, 49; mental disorders, 36–37; effectiveness in medicine, 42–43; mental health intervention studies, 43–46, 47–48; medical education, 50; medical education and communication skills, 55; doctor/patient relationship, 105; health care and inflation, 117; course offerings, 137. *See also* Economics
Counseling: medical students and stress, 184–85
Culture: somatization, 32; students and communication skills, 58; physicians and values, 73; ideology of science, 117, 213; differences and education, 169; medicine and Western thought, 202
Curriculum: behavioral and social sciences, 76–77; inflexibility and humanistic milieu, 97–98; courses to enhance attitudes and behavior, 136–40; reforms emphasizing problem-solving skills and clinical relevance, 140–48

Da Costa's syndrome: chest pain and psychiatric illness, 26–27

Dartmouth Medical School: videotaping and interviewing skills, 138; problem-based learning, 146–47; community-based learning experiences, 150–51, 152–53; faculty development, 164; innovative programs and alcoholism, 168–69
Daughters of Aesculapius: obstetrics and holistic medicine, 124–25
Death: pathological mourning, 7; students and communication, 66; oncology and stress, 184, 186, 191–92; religion and coping, 192
Dehumanization: medical schools, 98–99; brutalization and education, 204–207
Demography: medical students and communication, 60–62
Demoralization: women and stress in oncology, 191
Depersonalization: interpersonal aspects of patient care, 94–95; oncology and burnout syndrome, 185–86
Depression: grief and pathological mourning, 6, 7; bereavement and frequency, 10–11; symptoms of psychiatric illness, 26; medical students, 103; interns, 104; pediatric residents, 178; oncology house staff, 185, 193
Dermatology: symptoms and psychiatric illness, 28–29
Developing countries. *See* Third world
Disease: loss and onset, 10–13; choice of following bereavement, 13–14; age and onset, 14–16; separation and onset, 16–19; holistic view of in nineteenth century, 118–19
Dog: separation and disease onset, 19
Drugs: bereavement and tranquilizers, 11; psychotropic and management of psychiatric illness, 33; primary care physicians and mental disorders, 37
Dysmorphophobia: body image and psychiatric illness, 29

Economics: teaching hospital, 87–88, 99, 211; innovations in medical education, 130; community-based learning, 149. *See also* Cost
Education, medical: Nancy Roeske, 3; cost issues, 50; communication skills, 54–55, 68–70; environment and outcome, 84; Elizabeth Blackwell, 122; early female and emphasis on prevention, 123; history, 131–32; barriers to training of caringly competent physicians, 202–204; dehumanization and brutalization, 204–207; reasoning toward remedies, 209–14
———Innovation: programs and humanism, 108–109; approaches, 115; review of programs, 132–34; courses to enhance attitudes and behavior, 136–40; curricular reforms emphasizing problem-solving and

clinical relevance, 140–48; continuity of care and community-based learning experiences, 148–54; faculty development, 154–65; humanism, 165–66; surveys of outcomes, 166–67; limiting parameters, 167–68. *See also* Curriculum; Faculty; Medical schools

Elderly: institutions and deprivation, 10; bereavement and immune function, 15; psychiatric intervention and length of stay, 44–45; cost-offset effects of psychiatric intervention, 47–48

Emergencies: medical education, 86–87

Emory University: communication skills program, 65

Empathy: technology and communication, 56; burn-out and oncology house staff, 191

Endocrine system: age and disease onset, 15

Ethics: course offerings, 137

Face: pain and psychiatric illness, 26

Facts: values, 3–4; quantitative, 5

Faculty: education and communication skills, 68; selection criteria, 85; role-modeling, 89; class size, 99; research, 100; problem-based learning, 142; development and educational innovation, 154–65. *See also* Teachers and teaching

Family medicine: women doctors in nineteenth century, 120; patient-centered education, 150; competency-based faculty development, 162–63

Feelings: medical education, 109, 110

Food: allergies and psychiatric illness, 28

Fox, Renée: relationship with Roeske, 197–98

Functional disease. *See* Somatization

Funding: medical education, 89–90, 100–101; innovations in medical education, 130–31, 144; faculty development, 163

Gastrointestinal system: symptoms and psychiatric illness, 27–28

Gender: sex roles and communication patterns, 59–60; differentiation and medical culture, 126

Genetics: predisposition to disease, 13

GPEP Report: recommendations, 107, 200–201; learning, 132; process of education, 136

Grief: pathological reactions, 6–7

Gynecology: symptoms and psychiatric illness, 28

Harvard University: problem-based learning, 146; basic sciences and clinical learning, 170

Headache: psychiatric illness, 26

Health: human relationships, 5; effects of separation and loss, 5–7

Heart disease: bereavement and mortality

among widowers, 12; military medicine and psychiatric illness, 26–27

Hematology: community-based learning, 153

Hippocratic oath: role of physician, 74, 83, 94

Hormones: elderly and deprivation, 10

Hospital, teaching: environment of modern, 87–89, 99; nurses, 90; verbal abuse and humiliation of students, 100

Hospitalization: education and continuity of care, 148. *See also* Length of stay (LOS)

House staff. *See* Interns; Residents

Humaneness: physicians and body as machine, 4; evaluation of innovations in education, 134; patient and education, 136–37

Humanism: changing role of physician, 74; innovations in education, 165–66

Humanitarianism: educational experience and deterioration of student, 103

Humanities: education of physicians, 107

Hypertension: psychological makeup of patients, 14

Hyperventilation: psychiatric illness, 27

Hypochondriasis: psychiatric syndrome, 30

Hysteria: psychiatric illness, 26

Illness: onset of and loss, 10–13; biomedical and biopsychosocial models, 106–107

Immune system: loss and bereavement, 9–10; age and disease onset, 15; separation and disease onset, 18

Immunodeficiency: predisposition to disease, 13–14

Immunoglobulin: stress and levels, 10

Indiana University: curriculum, 76

Information: physician and learning skills, 78–79; students and stress, 97; faculty development, 164

Internal medicine: residencies and students, 88; competency-based faculty development, 163–65

Interns: psychological well-being, 103–104; stress and quality of care, 104–105; humanitarianism, 105; dehumanization and brutalization, 205–207

Interviews and interviewing: diagnosis of psychiatric syndromes, 30–31; students and communication skills, 57; Profile of Nonverbal Sensitivity (PONS), 65; importance and approach, 92–93; patients and depersonalization, 94–95; course offerings and innovation, 137–38; faculty development, 163

Irritable bowel syndrome: symptoms and psychiatric illness, 27–28

Jacobi, Mary Putnam: as teacher, 125

Johns Hopkins University: history of medical education, 131

Kellogg Foundation: funding of community-based learning, 153
Knowledge: physicians, 75–78; acquisition and students, 85–86

Language: developing countries and somatization, 32; house staff and world view, 212–13
Learning: physician and skills, 78; problem-based, 141–48
Length of stay (LOS): psychiatric comorbidity, 38–40, 42, 43; mental health treatment, 43–46; teaching hospitals, 99
Leukemia: psychobiology of loss in parents of victims, 9
Listening: doctors and communication skills, 54
Literature: image of physician, 73
Loss: personal attributes, 5; onset of illness and disease, 10–13. *See also* Bereavement; Separation

McMaster University: innovation in medical education, 132; integration of basic sciences and clinical practice, 141; problem-based learning, 142–43
Malpractice: communication, 62; physicians and values, 72; clinical teaching, 89; depersonalization of patient, 95
Medical College Admissions Test (MCAT): humanitarianism, 58
Medical schools: stress and information, 96–97; humanism and environment, 97–99, 110; female in nineteenth century, 125; rigidity and lack of integration, 169–70. *See also* Curriculum; Education, medical; Faculty
Medicine: values and human life, 4; biomedical and biopsychosocial models of illness, 106–107; nineteenth century view, 119; Western thought, 202–203; biological revolution, 210–11
Memorial Sloan-Kettering Cancer Center (MSKCC): stress intervention studies, 186–93
Men: medical students and communication, 59; stress and oncology, 191
Menopause: psychiatric morbidity, 28
Mental disorders (ADM): prevalence and cost, 36–37
Mental health: provision of services and cost of general medical care, 35–36; primary care physicians, 36–38; cost studies, 43–46; medical students, 103
Mice: separation and high blood pressure, 16–17
Michigan State University: minority students, 139; problem-based learning, 143–44, 160; faculty development, 154, 159–60

Moliere: image of physician, 73
Motherhood: women and medicine in nineteenth century, 119–20
Mount Sinai School of Medicine: humanistic medicine program, 109
Mourning: pathological grief reactions, 6–7; onset of disease and illness, 13
Myers-Briggs Personality Type Inventory: study skills programs, 138, 139

National Boards: innovative education, 167–68
National Institute of Mental Health (NIMH): provision of mental health services and cost of general medical care, 36
Network of Community-Oriented Educational Institutions for the Health Sciences: community-based learning, 153
New York Infirmary for Women and Children: preventive medicine, 123
New York State Health Department: house staff working hours, 102
Nucleoprotein: disturbances and separation, 19
Nurses: teaching hospital, 90; oncology and stress, 188

Obstetrics: female medical education in nineteenth century, 123–25
Oncology: community-based learning, 153; students, interns, and residents and stress, 183–93. *See also* Cancer
Organ system: medical education curriculum, 141

Pain: psychiatric illness, 26
Papalonicolou smears: cost-effectiveness, 42
Parasites: skin and psychiatric illness, 28
Parents: psychobiology of loss and leukemia, 9; students and communication skills, 65; role of pediatrician, 175–76
Patients: reasons for somatization, 31–32; student contact, 99; intern stress and quality of care, 104–105; humaneness and education, 136–37; continuity of care and medical education, 148–52; education and decision-making, 164; doctor as teacher, 164–65; oncology house staff and stress, 189, 190–91; difficult and house staff, 206–207
———Communication: dissatisfaction with physicans, 55–56, 95; house staff and non-verbal, 57–58; sick role experience, 58–59; medical students, 61
Pediatrician: role and adaptation, 175–76; house staff and stress, 176–80; resident adaptation program, 180–81
Personality: pediatrics and stress, 179; oncology and stress, 183–84, 192

Physician: compassion and body as machine, 4; patients and death or loss, 6; relationship with patient and psychiatric illness, 33; education and cost issues, 50; patient dissatisfaction and communication, 55–56; teaching patient to communicate, 69; attitudes, 72–75; knowledge, 75–78; skills required, 78–79; desirable characteristics, 84, 200; education in social sciences and humanities, 107. *See also* Primary care physicians

Physics: unity of intellectual efforts, 91

Placebo: therapeutic effect, 19; holistic medicine, 92

Policy: psychiatric intervention and cost of medical care, 48–49, 50

Power: physician and patient, 55, 57

Preston, Ann: as teacher, 126

Prevention: early female medical education, 123

Primary care physicians (PCP): mental health, 36–38; problem-based learning programs, 144, 145; community-based learning, 153–54

Profile of Nonverbal Sensitivity (PONS): interviewing, 65

Psychiatric illness: frequency and recognition, 25; presenting symptoms, 26–29; underlying syndromes, 29–31; management, 32–33. *See also* Somatization

Psychiatrists: contact with somatizing patients, 25; management of psychiatric illness, 33; communication skills, 63; integration of concepts of mind and brain, 203

Psychobiology: loss and separation in adults, 9–10

Psychology: psychogenic pain, 26, 30

Public health: medical school curriculum, 76

Pulse: separation and disturbances in rate, 17

Rats: stomach disease onset and age, 15
——Separation: experimental studies, 7–8; pulse rate, 17; sleep and temperature regulation, 17–18; gastric erosions, 18; immune function, 18; enzyme regulation, 18; growth, 18–19

Relationships, human: teaching importance of, 5; health, stress, and disease onset, 19; medical students, 102–103

Religion: oncology and stress, 191, 192

Research: design considerations, 46–47; faculty and teaching, 100; image of medical scientist, 121–22; Blackwell and education, 122; medical education and faculty development, 155, 160–61

Residents: training and stress, 101; working hours, 101–102; psychological well-being, 103–104; stress and oncology, 183–87; dehumanization and brutalization, 205–207

Respiration: symptoms and psychiatric illness, 27

Rhinoplasty: body image and psychiatric illness, 29

Robert Wood Johnson Foundation (RWJ): faculty development, 163

Roeske, Nancy: education of humane physicians, 3; Memorial Sloan-Kettering Cancer Center studies of stress, 193; relationship with Renée Fox, 197–98

Role models and modeling: Nancy Roeske and medical education, 3; teachers, 84; senior faculty, 89; students and humanistic care, 111; nineteenth-century female medical schools, 125

Rush Medical College: problem-based learning, 145–46

Science: medical school curriculum, 76; students and educational environment, 86; premedical curriculum, 96; culture and ideology, 117, 213; nineteenth-century view of medicine, 119; bacteriological revolution and medicine, 120–21; allopathic medicine, 131; problem-based learning, 145–46; molecular biology and medicine, 210–11

Self-understanding: programs and students, 138–40

Separation: experimental studies of health effects, 7–9; psychobiology of in adults, 9–10; disease onset, 16–19. *See also* Loss

Sexism: medical education and communication, 56, 59; gender-specific communication patterns, 59–60

Skin: psychiatric illness, 28–29

Sleep: disturbances and separation, 17–18

Smoking: bereavement, 11; Dartmouth Medical School, 152

Social sciences: medical school curriculum, 75–76; education of physicians, 107

Society of General Internal Medicine (SGIM): faculty development, 163–64

Somatization: definition, 24; studies of frequency, 25; patients and reasons, 31–32

Southern Illinois University: problem-based learning, 147

Specialization: role of physicians, 73; clinical teaching, 90; doctor/patient relationship, 106

State University of New York at Buffalo: faculty development and educational innovation, 154, 155–57, 159–60, 162, 164; success of innovation, 166–67

Stomach: age and disease onset, 15

Streptococcus: specific predisposition to particular disease, 13

Stress: residents and interns, 101; interns and quality of care, 104–105; house staff and reduction, 115; medical profession and education, 129–30; pediatric house staff, 176–80; resident adaptation program, 180–81; oncology students and house staff, 183–93; house staff and difficult patients, 206–207

Students, medical: environment and education, 85–86, 125; AIDS and prejudice, 95; changing population, 96; health, 102; personal relationships, 102–103; psychological well-being, 103; humane treatment, 110; models of humanistic care, 111; environment and attitudes, 129; programs for self-understanding and coping skills, 138–40; problem-based learning, 142–43; continuity of patient care and education, 148–52; stress and oncology, 183–86

———Communication: interviewing, 57; sociocultural context, 59–62; necessity for good, 62–63; suggested solutions, 63–68

Suicide: depression and bereavement, 11; interns, 104; medical students and stress, 185; oncology house staff, 193

Symptoms: physicians and frequency of somatic, 24; presenting of psychiatric illness, 26–28

Teachers and teaching: role models, 84; research funding and productivity, 100; medical education system, 110–11; training of caringly competent physicians, 207–209. *See also* Faculty

Technology: communication and empathy, 56; need for communication, 63; faculty and teaching, 85; medicine and sciences, 94; doctor/patient relationship, 105; computers and medical education, 136; faculty development, 164; cancer diagnosis and stress, 184

Temperature: regulation and separation, 17–18

Theology: unity of intellectual efforts, 91

Theory: values and facts, 4

Third world: language and somatization, 32; mental health care, 37; community-based learning, 153

Time: students and communication, 60; economics and teaching hospitals, 87–88 ·

Ulcers: genetics and predisposition, 13

Uncertainty: human condition and medical sciences, 204–205

United States: Briquet's syndrome, 30; cultural and socioeconomic patterns and educational reform, 133; teaching of clinical medicine, 211

U.S. Department of Health and Human Services (HHS): faculty development, 163

Universities: medical education and communication skills, 55; social sciences and curricula, 76–77; departments and educational philosophy, 84–85

University of Arizona: interviewing, 137

University of Illinois: orientation program, 139; faculty development, 154, 159, 161

University of Kansas Medical School: student attitudes and educational environment, 129

University of Maryland: prematriculation program, 139

University of Massachusetts School of Medicine: interviewing workshops, 137

University of Michigan Medical School: innovative educational program, 109

University of Missouri-Kansas City School of Medicine: communication skills program, 65

University of Nevada School of Medicine: academic support services, 139

University of New Mexico: problem-based learning, 144–45, 147, 148; community-based learning experiences, 151–52; faculty development, 164; students and socialization, 165, 168

University of Pennsylvania: faculty development, 154, 158

University of Saskatchewan: faculty development, 158–59

University of Southern California: faculty development, 154, 159

University of Texas: learning skills program, 139

Urinary 17-hydroxycorticosteroid (17-OHCS): psychobiology of loss in parents of leukemia victims, 9

Utrecht University School of Medicine: communication skills program, 64

Values: facts, 3–4, 5; humanism and physicians, 72

Venereal disease: genital symptoms and psychiatric illness, 28

Videotaping: interviewing skills, 137–38

Violence: physicians and communication, 66–67

Vivisection: Elizabeth Blackwell and education, 122

Vomiting: psychiatric illness, 27

Weight: growth and separation in rats, 18–19; brain function and separation in dogs, 19

Widows and Widowers: health and bereavement, 10, 12

Woman's Medical College of Pennsylvania: obstetrics education, 123–24; humanism of faculty, 126

Woman's Medical College of the New York Infirmary: obstetrics education, 124

Women: Briquet's syndrome, 30; psychiatric intervention and length of stay, 44–45; education and communication, 56, 59, 60–61; student population, 96; early physicians and humanitarianism, 115; patients and interviewing, 124; stress and oncology, 191. *See also* Gender; Sexism

World Wars: military medicine and psychiatric illness, 27

Zakrzewska, Marie: preventive medicine and placebos, 123